teach® yourself

reflexology
chris stormer

For over 60 years, more than 40 million people have learnt over 750 subjects the **teach yourself** way, with impressive results.

be where you want to be with **teach yourself**

For UK order enquiries: please contact Bookpoint Ltd., 130 Milton Park, Abingdon, Oxon OX14 4SB. Telephone: +44 (0) 1235 827720. Fax: +44 (0) 1235 400454. Lines are open from 09.00–18.00, Monday to Saturday, with a 24-hour message answering service. You can aso order through our website www.madaboutbooks.com.

For USA order enquiries: please contact McGraw-Hill Customer Services, PO Box 545, Blacklick, OH 43004-0545, USA. Telephone: 1-800-722-4726. Fax: 1-614-755-5645.

For Canada order enquiries: please contact McGraw-Hill Ryerson Ltd, 300 Water St, Whitby, Ontario L1N 9B6, Canada. Telephone: 905 430 5000. Fax: 905 430 5020.

Long-renowned as the authoritative source for self-guided learning – with more than 30 million copies sold worldwide – the *Teach Yourself* series includes over 300 titles in the fields of languages, crafts, hobbies, business, computing and education.

British Library Cataloguing in Publication Data: a catalogue record for this title is available from The British Library.

Library of Congress Catalog Card Number: on file

First published in UK 1996 by Hodder Headline Ltd., 338 Euston Road, London NW1 3BH.

First published in US 1996 by Contemporary Books, a Division of the McGraw-Hill Companies, 1 Prudential Plaza, 130 East Randolph Street, Chicago IL. 60601 USA.

The 'Teach Yourself' name is a registered trade mark of Hodder & Stoughton Ltd.

Artwork by Lori Marilyn Hughes

Typeset by Transet Limited, Coventry, England.
Printed in Great Britain for Hodder & Stoughton Educational, a division of Hodder Headline Ltd., 338 Euston Road, London NW1 3BH by Cox & Wyman Ltd., Reading, Berkshire.

Impression number   7 6 5 4 3 2 1
Year   2007 2006 2005 2004 2003

iii

contents

acknowledgements

My sincere thanks to the publishers, Hodder Headline, for inviting me to write this book. I have thoroughly enjoyed the opportunity of sharing knowledge of reflexology in a slightly different way from my previous books.

As always, none of this would have been possible without the incredible love and support of my family, particularly my wonderful man, John Fryer, my two outstanding sons, Andrew and David, and my amazing parents, Dick and Daphne Corner. The depth of my affection and appreciation can never be adequately expressed.

My gratitude to **all** tutors, therapists and students of RASA worldwide for enriching my life, as well as generously sharing individual expertise and universal knowledge, much of which has been passed on in this book to assist others to help themselves.

To the readers, if it were not for your enlightened desire for personal development, books like this would not be possible.

May abundant happiness and ultimate fulfilment be yours.

Running Water, my guide – Thank You!

Teach Yourself Reflexology is an easy-to-follow guide to a natural, effective and safe form of healing that has stood the test of time and continues to be everybody's birthright. This book includes brief explanations of its background and origins, as well as of how it works and what to expect during and after the massage. In this way fascinating insight can be gained into this ancient therapy.

Simple step-by-step instructions of reflexology guide you reassuringly through the massage of both feet, section by section, as follows:

- the toes to ease the mind
- the toe necks to open the avenues of two-way expression
- the balls of the feet to pacify the emotions
- the insteps for inner harmony
- the heels for personal growth and development
- the corresponding parts for overall well-being.

Clear illustrations accompany the instructions to facilitate understanding. From this basis and with experience, comprehension and confidence, you will be able to expand and develop your own unique approach.

Reflexology is exceptionally accommodating and it does not matter if, initially, attempts are slow, cumbersome, inaccurate or confused. The body naturally compensates for any perceived inadequacy.

It is impossible to cause harm, even in inexperienced hands.

Furthermore, an understanding of how transient thoughts and inner emotions are constantly mirrored through the ever-changing characteristics of the feet will dispel any fear, especially when it comes to massaging the feet of temporarily imbalanced, unwell souls.

The more common ailments that respond particularly well to reflexology massage are listed to show how a change of mind and pacification of unsettled emotions can transform an individual from being fraught, uptight and uneasy into feeling totally relaxed, flexible and energized.

Reflexology is truly remarkable in the way it encourages everybody to help themselves to a more fulfilling, rewarding and better way of life. The marvel of being able to mould and create a stunning new reality continues to amaze the recipients of this sensitive, yet incredibly effective form of massage of the feet, no matter how skeptical they may initially be!

We all possess a very great power – the ability to heal ourselves.

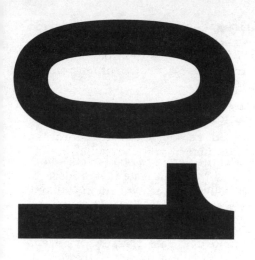

01

an explanation
of reflexology

In this chapter you will unearth:
- how reflexology is an ancient and natural form of healing that has stood the test of time for many centuries.

A general overview

Reflexology is the firm, but gentle massage that coaxes reflexes in both feet to:

- ease tension in the physical body
- quieten the mental chatter
- soothe the emotions
- reconnect at soul level.

By alerting latent healing abilities within the body, reflexology assists in creating a healthy, harmonious state that is ideal for the efficient and effective physical, mental, emotional and spiritual functioning of the whole.

This natural form of healing has stood the test of time as an ancient, non-invasive, simple and safe therapy. It is still responsible for remarkable reactions experienced worldwide today.

Reflexology arouses or soothes to fine-tune corresponding parts of the body through the perceptive massage of reflexes in the feet. These reflexes accurately and precisely reflect bodily parts, organs and glands in miniature. Touching specific reflexes on the feet can, therefore, evoke a favourable, involuntary reflex response in the related part of the body.

> *Feet also explicitly reflect the state of the mind, body and soul through the condition and texture of their soles.*

The sudden surge of vibrant energy generated by reflexology massage rejuvenates the physical body, flushes away emotional impediments and establishes a state of inner peace so that a natural state of health can either be regained and/or retained.

For the healthy person, reflexology offers:

- a pleasant form of deep relaxation
- relief from fear, anxiety and frustration
- rejuvenation that re-energizes mind, body and soul
- increased vitality and confidence
- improved quality of sleep
- trust in personal attributes and those of others
- prolonged acute concentration
- a feeling of incredible well-being
- restored balance

- a sense of wholeness
- a more fulfilling and rewarding experience of life and health
- the courage to cope beneficially with perceived adversity
- the confidence to express one's truth openly with pure love and honesty
- an opportunity for personal transformation, growth and individual development.

For the less healthy, reflexology:

- eases uneasiness within
- relieves and deals with the root cause of dis-content
- counteracts fatigue
- soothes nervousness, worry and fear
- eases aches, pains and dis-comfort
- alleviates distress
- reduces tension by relaxing the musculature
- improves circulation
- cleanses the whole of threatening substances and impurities
- stimulates hypo-active, sluggish, inactive areas
- calms hyperactive, over-productive parts.

There are many advantages to learning reflexology.

- Anyone and everyone from toddlers onwards can do it, provided there is an interest.
- It can be administered at any time, or in any situation, since the only essential requirements are the hands of the masseur and the feet of the recipient.
- Aacademic achievements are not a pre-requisite.
- Medical knowledge is useful but not essential.
- Only the feet are exposed, reducing embarrassment, self-consciousness and possible vulnerability.
- Painful bodily parts are left undisturbed, yet relief can still be obtained by massaging the related reflexes in the feet.
- With less skin surface on the feet than on the body, a more thorough and precise treatment is possible.

Acquiring knowledge of reflexology is a fascinating, enjoyable and rewarding journey. Although there is no right or wrong way to apply this technique, it does help to have a basic understanding of certain applied principles to facilitate its application.

The reflexology massage generally takes about an hour, yet its effects last much longer, with favourable reactions, even from cynics. This is because reflexology is one of the most encompassing and holistic disciplines of healing known to humankind.

Health and healing are only two feet away!

History and background

The practice and knowledge of reflexology has been passed from generation to generation for centuries. When humans first 'set foot' on earth, their soles were naturally stimulated every time they 'put their foot down' on the undulating ground until such time that sandals and shoes were introduced, when the barrier created increasingly diminished the inborn sensitivity of feet. This is where reflexology stepped in!

Feet have always played a vital role in the journey through life and have contributed greatly to the progress and advancement of humanity.

Throughout history, feet have symbolized mobility, security and the foundation of mind, body and soul.

According to Greek legend, feet symbolized the soul, with any lameness being perceived as weakness of spirit.

The ancient Egyptians used to peel away the 'soles' of the feet during mummification, to liberate the 'soul' from its physical bondage and commitment to earth.

Witches, on being declared guilty, were immediately raised from the ground, to sever their contact with Mother Earth, since it was believed that they absorbed their mystical powers via the feet.

Until AD 200, many flocked to the Delphi health resort in Greece to relax in the sacred waters of the hydrotherapy pools. Before retiring to a sleep temple, reflexology and body massage were administered to evoke memories and foresight through dreams. The interpretation of these visions provided guidance and direction on their continued journey through life.

According to Japanese mythology, there was once a wise old soul called Otou, who, when questioned about his incredible healing powers, would say:

'See to the feet, my friend, and you have seen to the body.' 'I do not understand', bewildered investigators would protest. Otou gently replied, 'Your understanding will never be enough. See to the feet, that is all that is required.'

Otou was aware that feet reveal the mind, body and soul on every level.

There are many references to feet in the Bible, which mentions the symbolic ritual of welcome and purification through anointing, washing and massaging feet. Reflexology is a furtherance of this sacred act of acceptance since it encourages internal cleansing for purity throughout.

Kissing and worshipping the feet of divine or eminent souls is still a sign of respect that was, for centuries, evident in cultures worldwide. It is now mainly practised in certain rural parts of India, where youngsters still kiss the feet of their parents as a sign of love and appreciation.

Today many seek the opportunity to glimpse or touch the feet of devout, spiritual men in India, such as Sai Baba. To do so is believed to attain inner peace and personal enlightenment. Devotees also gather dust from the Baba's footprints or drink water that has been poured over their feet to enhance the illumination and evoke inner serenity.

For centuries, countless people have found relief from extreme discomfort, by turning to reflexology, when all else failed.

One of them was the twentieth President of the United States of America, President Garfield (1831–1881), who suffered excruciating pain after an assassination attempt. He received endless types of treatment but it was only when he turned to reflexology that he gained increased comfort and relief.

Reflexology is a self-help therapy that has, and still is providing natural healing worldwide, regardless of skin colour, religious conviction or social belief system. Its simplicity has to date demeaned its remarkable effectiveness in harmonizing the whole, which is why reflexology is now being reinstated as an all-encompassing healing therapy that keeps individuals in 'good working order'.

> *Feet represent our roots and foundations. If restricted, the individual's potential is limited. Once liberated, the individual is free to venture forth unimpeded.*

Complementing one another: modern medicine and reflexology

Orthodox medicine, at only 300 years old, is extremely young compared to complementary healing methods, such as reflexology, which dates back many centuries. Through medical research, however, natural forms of healing have gained greater insight and comprehension of the anatomical, physiological and pathological structure as well as the working of the mind and body. Through this understanding ancient healing methods have made remarkable advancements. By continually adapting and adjusting their approach they have been able to keep pace with the ever-changing and progressive needs of modern society.

Interestingly, the expansive development and sophistication of the mind is repeatedly reflected through the on-going physical enlargement of the body and feet. Individuals are becoming increasingly comfortable with taking up more space and are more confident about making a greater impression and larger impact on life.

Hippocrates, the acknowledged Father of Medicine, believed that emotions, responsible for the mind's disposition and the ever-changing physical condition, could be detected through fluctuations in body humours. In this way, the most appropriate remedy could be determined.

The state of the body certainly reflects the content or dis-content of the mind:

- health is the natural state of ease and inner peace
- dis-ease outwardly reflects inner conflict or turmoil.

The balance between health and dis-ease, nonetheless, is easily toppled when there is an unhealthy obsession with tempting aspects within the physical, materialistic world, which can deprive the soul of ultimate fulfilment on earth. If this leads to an impoverished self-esteem and self-worth, then it is more likely to manifest physically through perceived deprivation, self-criticism and personal denial.

This is why overall harmony and health are only possible when there is complete enrichment on all levels of mind, body and soul.

Modern technology is incredible because individuals are now liberated from mundane tasks, and have more time for creative worthwhile pursuits that can be extremely satisfying and exceptionally fulfilling, which in turn provides greater opportunity for on-going personal growth and self-development.

If these opportunities are overlooked or ignored, however, then varying degrees of discontent, frustration and bewilderment disrupt the whole, leading to flagellating mind-talk that is upsetting and increases the possibility of dis-ease, arising from uneasiness within.

Modern medicine effectively caters for bodily and intellectual needs by offering solutions that relieve physical pain and mental dis-comfort. When used advantageously, these welcome stepping-stones can soothe the symptoms of dis-ease long enough for changes to take place on an emotional and spiritual level, which should make one feel much better.

A complete shift of mindset and change of attitude are essential for total relief from discomfort and illness, since life is the product of personal perceptions.

For example, on-going irritability either manifests in the form of skin rashes or increased mucus production or hypersensitivity, and it will continue to do so until a more tolerant or less benevolent outlook replace this tetchiness.

Placebos, tablets without drug content, can also be effective antidotes especially when administered with a conviction that is so profoundly convincing that the recipient has a complete shift of consciousness.

Whatever the mind believes becomes the body's reality.

Even though it is not possible to re-align broken bones through reflexology, it is possible, through relaxation, to ease discomfort and accelerate the healing process by creating a conducive and tranquil environment.

Reflexology encourages natural health by healing mind, body and soul, at a subconscious level, without having to evoke or stir past traumatic memories, which avoids having to go through any further emotional havoc and distress.

Modern medical knowledge gives reflexology and other forms of complementary healing the incentive to take healing a step further. Just as symptoms of dis-ease reflect the state of mind, so it is that the characteristics of the feet accurately display the root cause of unsettling circumstances long before they manifest as dis-ease in the body. Through greater understanding of specific individual needs, the healing session can be adapted accordingly.

Reflexology and modern medicine, when used beneficially together, are a dynamic combination.

A more wholistic approach to healing is being adopted by medical professionals worldwide, with many now prescribing reflexology, along with more conventional treatments, to accelerate the recovery process. Results to date have been phenomenal. The combination of reflexology and modern medicine has the advantage of integrating ancient knowledge and wisdom with modern, sophisticated technology, so that everybody can benefit from both modalities.

> *Competition and comparisons are futile because each individual is meant to be unique for the on-going exchange and sharing of extraordinary ideas and unusual concepts.*

Other forms of complementary healing

Natural healing mediums provide an array of therapies and remedies on which the mind, body and soul can thrive.

The **Alexander technique** realigns bodily posture, which balances the musculature and re-energizes the whole. Reflexology enhances the effect of this procedure by easing tension and relaxing the muscles.

Aromatherapy uses the evocative sense of aromatic smell, usually through bodily massage. Massaging feet with exquisite oils, either during or after reflexology, steps up the healing process. Try this popular combination of:

> Juniper to detoxify
> Bergamot to calm the nerves
> Neroli to boost self-confidence
> Ylang-Ylang to heighten the senses

Colour healing balances the finely tuned body by equalizing personal vibrations. Application of colour through visualization during a reflexology massage, advantageously alters the overall tone of mind, body and soul (see Appendix II).

Crystals and other gems have potent healing properties. Holding a rose quartz loosely in each hand during reflexology encourages self-acceptance and fills the whole with renewed vibrancy, especially when the stones are gently placed on the solar plexus reflexes (pages 130–1) at the end of the massage.

Flower Remedies are natural extracts from the plant kingdom, which taken orally calm persistent threatening thoughts and adjust mood swings. Combined with reflexology, soul-destroying cycles become more manageable. Keep a bottle of Rescue Remedy handy at all times just in case of extreme emotional distress whilst massaging the feet.

Herbs have numerous remedial qualities because they are a natural source of energy, which complements reflexology beautifully in preserving health.

Homeopathy and naturopathy are plant derivatives that alleviate dis-ease naturally. They help to prolong the empowering effect of reflexology, particularly when used between sessions.

Music rearranges body particles through sound vibrations, which, when integrated with reflexology, can be exceptionally therapeutic since the basic structure is rearranged to recreate inner harmony (see Appendix III).

- Mozart's music is rich in high frequencies, which fills the whole with vibrancy and enthusiasm
- Gregorian chants create inner sacredness
- dolphin and whale music calms and reassures, especially pregnant ladies, children, dis-eased and unconscious souls.

Reiki shifts and balances bodily vibrations by directing life forces to areas that lack energy and vitality. The effect is magnified on all levels when combined with reflexology.

Shiatsu, acupressure and acupuncture clear energy pathways for the penetration of natural life forces to all bodily cells.

Everybody and everything in life is essentially neutral. It is the intent of actions, interactions and reactions that makes a world of difference.

02

the role of reflexology

In this chapter you will discover:
- that reflexology enhances self-awareness
- how reflexology gives body, mind and soul new freedom, co-ordination and energy.

Ease or disease

Every individual has a unique approach to life, which determines whether emotions are in tune or in conflict with the natural flow of energy. This creates the ease or dis-ease of mind, body and soul.

A healthy person is calm, yet wakes up energized, enjoys any challenge that comes their way, continually looks for worthwhile opportunities to grow and develop, enthuses about everything they do and appreciates the gift and fullness of life. This is known as 'having a life' and the true art of 'living'.

Whilst a wholesome attitude exudes well-being, dis-ease is the product of constant complaints, on-going criticism and general discomfort from trying to live up to ridiculous expectations. As the body becomes isolated from its soul's purpose, the individual becomes intensely frustrated, bewildered, doubtful, unhappy and emotionally lonely.

Conforming to limited, often outdated and unreasonable belief systems robs people of their individuality and denies them of numerous opportunities to realize and utilize their own unique talents. The subsequent build up of resentment then becomes discernible as physical tension, which:

- hampers personal progress
- interferes with individual performance
- causes overreaction to minor, seemingly insignificant, situations
- results in misplaced anger or impatience
- increases or decreases the appetite
- leads to the abuse of
  - alcohol to drown one's sorrows
  - food to cover up the true self or provide protection against perceived maltreatment
  - tobacco to form a smokescreen that conceals soulful emotions
  - drugs to desensitize personal turmoil.

At the core of a dis-eased person is a potentially healthy soul. Being pushed to the limits forces them to think again to reassess their situation and strategy in life, with the innate knowledge that there is always plenty of room for betterment.

Physical symptoms of distress signal inner unhappiness and dissatisfaction.

Consciously or unconsciously there is an inherent desire within everybody to be whole, healthy and balanced which is immediately disturbed whenever one's authenticity is threatened. This can 'knock an individual off their feet', veering them way off into the extremes of the unknown, which is made worse by increased vulnerability from the belief that one is under attack for not being good enough.

Sickness is sometimes the only thing that will make us wake up to who we are and stimulate the deep change required within.

'Finding one's feet' again, through the use of inner resources and internal strength, allows rediscovery of profound and amazing aspects of oneself. In the process of 'getting back on one's feet', it is possible to step ahead with even greater understanding and insight for the next leg of the journey of self-discovery through life.

The body's language is vividly and accurately reflected through the ever-changing characteristics of the feet. The condition of the soles reflects the state of the soul in the following ways:

- *ill-at-ease*: tense and uptight
- *injured*: dents and/or various shades of blue to black revealing hurt pride and bruised feelings
- *upset*: overall lack composure
- *invalid*: devoid of strength and energy
- *off colour*: drained of vibrancy and predominantly white
- *weak*: lack substance
- *troubled*: wrinkled and lined skin on the feet
- *disabled*: unable to move ahead due to some perceived impediment or disadvantage
- *distorted*: contorted from trying to fit into unsuitable and unfashionable belief systems.

Although the underlying circumstances of dis-ease differ from one person to the next, the body has marvellous natural recuperative abilities that come to the fore, especially in the healthy and relaxed environment created through the massage of the feet.

Healthy people feed their minds with loving thoughts that clear the pathway to success. Each day is then seen to be an opportunity to do something worthwhile, with limitless enthusiasm and ingenuity.

Just the fact that we are living is important!

Defusing distress

Distress causes the inadequate functioning or breakdown of bodily parts, which could lead to any of the following possible outcomes:

- **ulcers** from frustration that eats away at oneself
- **hypertension** due to pressure from unresolved emotional conflicts
- **heart dis-ease** arising from:
  - lack of pure love for oneself and others
  - hardening of the heart in favour of acquiring material possessions
  - fear of not being good enough, which squeezes and constricts it causing pain
  - constant criticism of everybody and everything
- **strokes** from relentlessly being controlled or from trying to gain the upper hand
- **kidney failure** from overwhelming disappointment and disillusionment.

Massaging the feet directs life force energies along natural energy pathways within the body to unleash energy knots and flush out emotional congestion, which is the physical manifestation of harmful thought patterns.

Clearing impediments may cause initial exhaustion and lethargy as the body reactivates its natural healing resources, which are strong enough to overcome any symptom, no matter how minor or serious.

Without pressure, the relaxed mind, body and soul can function effectively and efficiency due to the renewed surge of vital energy that invigorates the whole.

Reflexology's history of combating distress and disease worldwide is impressive. The widespread incidence of regaining and retaining health could lead to an epidemic of well-being, which would mean a phenomenal decrease of all illnesses, as well as a drop in medical and hospital expenses.

> *That which we release heals us, that which we restrain inhibits our personal development.*

Feet!

Feet provide a solid foundation and flexible mobility for personal growth and individual development. Like roots, they afford security and stability, but have the added advantage of being able to adapt to the unexpected 'ups and downs' of ongoing experiences that are continually encountered on the journey through life.

Fear, uncertainty and anxiety 'root feet to the ground' or 'allow the grass to grow under the feet'. These rigid, unhappy, insecure soles continually 'test the way' due to being 'unsure of their footing'. This makes for an arduous and heavy going trip.

Secure, content people, on the other hand, enjoy 'standing on their own two feet' and 'with a foot in the door' know that they can 'step ahead with confidence' in a relaxed and happy manner. With 'a spring in their step' and natural flexibility, these souls readily adjust to the unexpected twists and turns around many corners.

The frequent use of the words 'foot' or 'feet' in describing a person's standing or situation in life is symbolic, reiterating their importance as some of the more commonly used sayings suggest:

- land on one's feet: secure a fortunate position
- find one's feet: settle down
- put the best foot forward: make a good impression
- put one's foot down: take a firm stand
- put one's foot in it: make a faux pas
- trample under foot: oppress or treat with contempt
- be on good footing: be on friendly terms.

Feet provide a basic understanding of individual requirements. When relaxed, the rest of the body has the potential to be healthy. They also display personal talents that, when realized, can make a world of difference. This is where reflexology plays a big role.

> *Our feet reveal the story of our life.*

Who benefits from reflexology?

Anyone and everyone can benefit from reflexology's amazing ability to harmonize all bodily systems. It effectively enhances the functioning of mind, body and soul. As a relaxation technique, reflexology:

- reassures the body
- eases muscular tension
- creates space for healing to occur
- naturally stimulates sluggish, hypo-active glands and organs
- soothes over-excited, hyperactive bodily parts.

With gentle, sensitive application, it is impossible to cause harm with reflexology since it is a non-invasive therapy.

Be wary, however, of massaging the feet of a deep vein thrombosis sufferer, who experiences excruciating pain from a blood clot, generally in the legs. This is because, as the muscles relax their grip on the circulatory system, the blood clot may become dislodged and may then travel to the brain or heart, with the remote possibility of a stroke or heart attack. Although there has been no report of such an occurrence, it is still advisable to be cautious.

Reflexology is particularly effective during:

- pregnancy (see also pages 167–71)
    - the mother-to-be enjoys on-going energy and inner peace
    - the relaxed womb expands more easily to accommodate the baby
    - the calm environment ensures the healthy growth and development of new life
    - foetal movement within the uterus is unhindered
    - nourishment of mother and baby is ensured through lively circulation
    - vital energy abounds throughout
    - there is a stronger bond of trust and unconditional love for one another.

- childhood

Babies and children are so finely tuned into parental thoughts and feelings, that they subconsciously manifest these through their own state of health, generally before the parent is aware of what is really going on.

- makes them less sensitive
- soothes hyperactivity
- calms and reassures
- increases harmony and ease within the home
- strengthens physical, emotional and spiritual ties
- encourages self-acceptance
- permits individual growth and development.

- adolescence
  - balances hormonal production and distribution for inner harmony
  - encourages a more trusting and honest relationship within oneself and amongst others
  - aids confidence
  - provides the impetus to step into adulthood with increased tolerance and poise.

- adult years
  - keeps mind, body and soul in good working condition
  - provides faith in life's processes
  - wrinkles of concern are less likely to leave their mark
  - takes a burden off mind, body and soul
  - releases weighty issues, making the body less prone to sagging
  - encourages a more lenient, open-minded attitude
  - eases self-induced pressure
  - minimizes the damaging effect of distress, fear and anxiety.

- golden years
  - prevents mind, body and soul from withering and wasting away
  - injects the whole with renewed enthusiasm for life
  - provides a meaningful purpose to life
  - alerts the mind
  - improves concentration
  - preserves the body by replacing worn-out cells with new, healthy, vibrant cells.

- during illness
  - meets the need for touch
  - eases ill health, vulnerability and defencelessness
  - soothes distress

- – relieves symptoms of uneasiness
- – eliminates harmful substances and destructive emotions
- – makes space for the development of healthy, rejuvenated cells
- – calms the mind, relaxes the body and reassures the soul.
- within the family unit
  - – bridges the gap between the generations
  - – strengthens the bond between all family members
  - – encourages acceptance and understanding of personal attributes
  - – creates respect and understanding for individuality.

Health and healing are the natural state of well being when there is overall unity and harmony through peace of mind, a relaxed body and a contented soul.

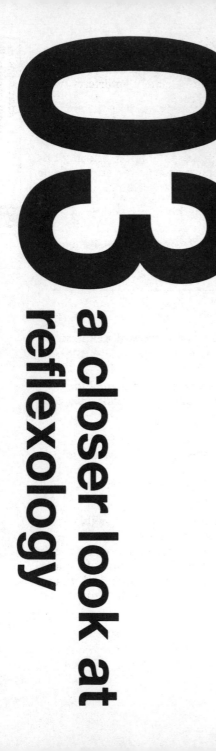

03

a closer look at reflexology

In this chapter you will find out:
- how reflexology relaxes the body for it be an effective channel through which the fine vibrations of healing can travel.

How reflexology works

Protracted fear, anxiety and distrust cause uneasiness throughout, which causes tension that immediately interferes with natural bodily functions and processes.

The greater the uneasiness, the greater the fraughtness and the more damaging the interference.

Distressing thoughts devastate and alarm the body, causing it to defend itself instinctively and prepare its cells for an attack or from any form of perceived adversity that seemingly threatens its well-being.

- the musculature becomes up-tight
- tense, contracted muscles clamp down on the internal structures
- this reduces the amount of space in which body parts can function
- the subsequent rigidity inhibits mobility
- areas become depleted of blood
- affected bodily cells are starved of nutritional sustenance
- these deprived cells are then denied the opportunity to grow and develop to their full capacity
- potentially dangerous toxic substances accumulate and become trapped by the narrowed lumen or flaccid veins and lymphatic vessels
- body, mind and soul become burdened.

Uneasiness of the mind is displayed through symptoms of distress and dis-ease. This is the body's way of attracting attention in the hope that beneficial steps are taken to change the frightful and fear-filled situation.

Pain is the desperate plea from distressed, deprived cells within the body. It is their way of begging the brain to let go and ease tension so that vital substances can get through to nourish them. If the situation is not alleviated through relaxation, fear and misunderstanding of the pain cause further panic and strain, which can then affect neighbouring or related cells causing the dis-ease and pain to spread.

Any prolonged tension denies affected cells space, nutrients and vital life forces, which means that they are more likely to malfunction and, eventually, become malformed, a condition more commonly known as cancer.

Reflexology is a relaxation technique that dissipates tension, relieves pressure and ultimately disperses dis-ease. As the muscles relax their tight grip on the musculature the following occurs:

- increased elasticity allows for greater flexibility and mobility
- the ability to naturally expand and contract improves body functioning
- the boosted blood flow generously replenishes all bodily cells
- the well-nurtured cells now have space to function and rejuvenate themselves
- potentially harmful substances are eliminated
- a weight is lifted off the mind, body and soul
- an ideal environment is created for the efficient functioning of the whole
- good health is promoted.

Reflexology soothes from the inside out and is an impressive antidote to distress. The recipient drifts into a deeply relaxing and blissful state of alpha consciousness, the tranquil phase that naturally occurs between wakefulness and sleep. The mind, body and soul are able to take advantage of this autonomy to regroup and fully recuperate.

This is possible because every second, billions of new cells are formed throughout the mind and body for on-going efficiency. If there is no meddling with this amazing rejuvenation process, ageing is no longer a possibility!

A relaxed body naturally re-energizes itself through the absorption of abundant universal energy, which it obtains from two main sources, the sun and the earth:

- hair on the head and covering the body acts as antennae and absorbs the vibrant, positive, light energies of Father sun
- the soles of the feet draw in the solid, dark, negative energies of Mother earth.

These energies surround and penetrate the body and, in so doing, replenish the whole with renewed and essential vitality. The resulting vibrancy within the various organs and glands bounces back to the body's surface and is reflected through the changing characteristics of the body and feet.

Any interference to this natural sequence distresses the body, and this is immediately mirrored in the feet as follows:

- rigidity indicates extreme insecurity and uncertainty
- hardness covers up or conceals vulnerability
- flaccidity reveals perceived personal deprivation or lack of inner substance
- weakness occurs when there is a lack of inner strength and on-going resourcefulness
- poor stature shows exhaustion from not getting ahead.

Heavy, unhappy thoughts, from doubt and uncertainty, weigh greatly on the mind and body, with similar heaviness and lifelessness being reflected in the feet. Reflexology encourages the subconscious release of these burdensome notions and emotions, whilst, at the same time, putting stored beliefs and anxious memories into perspective so that they are no longer an apparent threat to personal well-being.

A relaxed physical body is able to let go of physical restraints that have a repercussive effect on the mental, emotional and spiritual aspects of the whole. The individual consequently feels better, can think more clearly and can get on with enjoying life to the full.

All perceived adversities, large or small, can be a destructive force OR advantageously used for even greater personal growth and development.

Position of the reflexes

The relay of reflexology from generation to generation over many centuries has inevitably meant that the perceived reflex positions have been influenced by individual perception and interpretation, which has led to slight alterations of their actual positions.

This has resulted in an assortment of foot charts, which although basically the same, do show differing reflexes, especially of the spine, ears, eyes, heart, breasts and knees.

Many organs, glands and parts do, however, overlap in the body, which means that there are many reflexes in any one part of the feet. This is particularly relevant when it comes to the nerves, blood and lymph vessels since they infiltrate the whole body. Also bone and muscle reflexes are present throughout because they provide the basic infrastructure of the whole.

Furthermore there is more than one way to access a reflex. A primary reflex provides direct access, whilst a secondary reflex approaches the area more indirectly. For example, the breasts are reflected directly onto the balls of the feet, but are still accessible through the secondary or indirect reflexes, which are situated directly opposite on the tops of both feet (Figure 1).

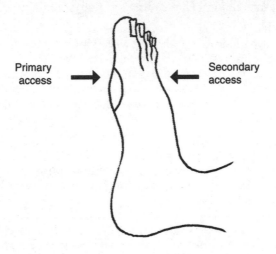

Primary access   Secondary access

figure 1 primary and secondary breast reflexes

It is possible to see how perfectly all bodily parts are reflected by simply visualizing a miniature version of the body's anatomy on the feet (Figure 2, pages 23–24).

- each foot represents half the body
- the front of the body is mirrored onto the soles of the feet
- the back of the body is depicted on the tops of the feet
- the right side of the body is reflected onto the right foot
- the left foot corresponds with the left side of the body.

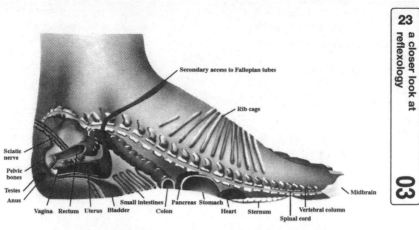

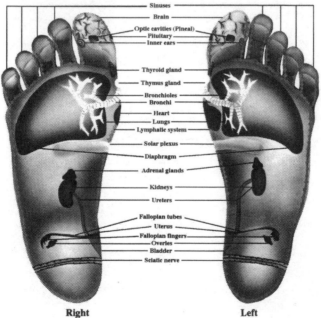

figure 2 reflection of bodily parts in miniature on the feet

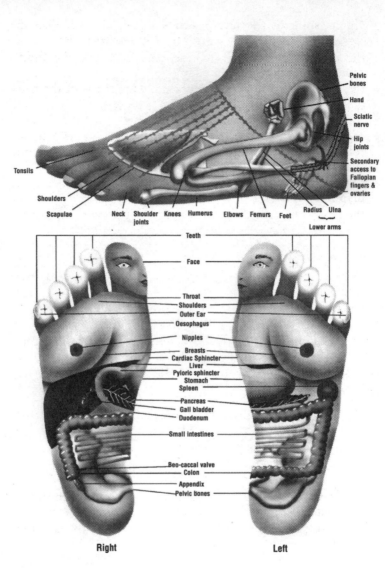

Pelvic bones
Hand
Sciatic nerve
Hip joints
Secondary access to Fallopian fingers & ovaries

Tonsils
Shoulders
Scapulae
Neck
Shoulder joints
Knees
Humerus
Elbows
Femurs
Feet
Radius
Ulna
Lower arms

Teeth
Face
Throat
Shoulders
Outer Ear
Oesophagus
Nipples
Breasts
Cardiac Sphincter
Liver
Pyloric sphincter
Stomach
Spleen
Pancreas
Gall bladder
Duodenum
Small intestines
Beo-caccal valve
Colon
Appendix
Pelvic bones

Right

Left

With the soles of the feet placed side by side, visualize the following bodily parts, on a substantially smaller scale:

- the cushioned toe pads represent the face and the multi-dimensional aspects of the brain
- the big toes, placed together, resemble the shape of the head and face
- toe necks mirror the neck and throat
- together the balls of the feet form the chest and breast reflexes, with their solidarity resembling the hard bony ribcage
- the domes at the bases of the balls of both feet are the diaphragm reflexes
- the fleshy insteps represent the soft fleshy abdominal cavity
- the dense heels are solid like the bony pelvis.

The accuracy of this is so great that:

- there is a corresponding gap, or hollow, where any body part is missing or has been removed
- when scar tissue has formed there is a matching hardness
- extra bones and organs rebound in the reflected position
- crushed bone feels shattered, splintered or gritty in the feet.

Back and limb reflexes on the outer edges of the feet (figure 3)

- the solid upper surfaces of both feet reflect the back of the body and carry the marks and impressions of:
  - all that is going on 'behind one's back'
  - events that have been 'placed in the background'
  - that which an individual has 'turned their back on'
- below each little toe, on top of the feet, are prominent bones that match the upper arm socket
- bony protrusions halfway down the outer edges on each foot correspond to the elbow joints
- the outer ankle-bones represent the external edges of the hip-bones
- limb reflexes can be distinguished by various corresponding bone formations.

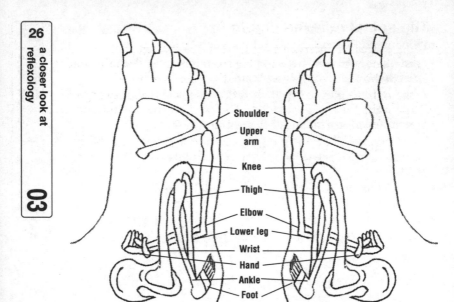

figure 3 back and limb reflexes on the outer edges of both feet

Back and limb reflexes on the soles of both feet (figure 4)

- the limbs are also reflected onto the soles of both feet with the body depicted in a seated position with both knees bent.

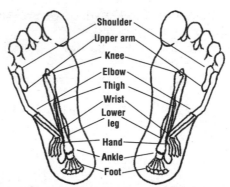

figure 4 limb reflexes on the soles of both feet

The spinal reflexes (figure 5)

- the ridges of intervallic bone that stretch along the inside edges of both feet, from the big toe joints to beneath the inner ankle-bones, represent the spinal vertebrae reflexes
- the right side of the spine is reflected along the inner edge of the right foot whilst the left side of the vertebral column is reflected along the inner edge of the left foot.

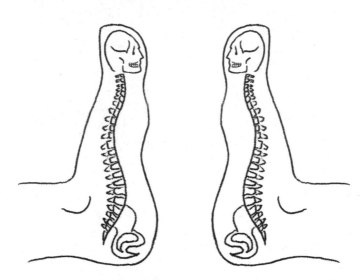

figure 5 divided spinal reflexes on both feet

Visualizing the various bodily reflexes on the feet assists the reflexology massage considerably.

Inner and outer aspects of the feet (figure 6)

For the purpose of this book:

- the inner edges refer to reflexes on the medial aspect of the feet and toes, on the sides where the big toes are situated
- the outer edge refers to reflexes on the lateral parts, on the sides where the little toes are positioned.

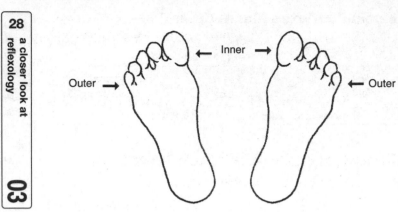

figure 6 inner and outer aspects of the feet

The effects of reflexology

Recipients generally feel fantastic after receiving reflexology! They are more alert, completely rejuvenated and enormously refreshed yet, at the same time, very relaxed and extremely content. Their feet tingle with delight as they move ahead with a 'spring in their step'.

During reflexology tension is released, allowing circulation within the relaxed blood vessels to become positively lively, which encourages the more effective and efficient distribution of nutrients and vital life-forces throughout. Meanwhile, the elimination of toxic, wasteful substances becomes easier in this mellow environment. The resultant detoxification is synonymous with letting go of menacing, worthless emotions that have the potential to be destructive and soul destroying.

Reflexology immediately dispenses with any unwanted contents to avoid any further impediment to personal growth and self-development. Exoneration of emotional burdens lightens the mind, body and soul, and creates ample room for inner peace and homoeostasis.

Conditions are then ideal for natural, efficient functioning, physically, mentally, emotionally and spiritually. On a quantum level, the body's energy fields are totally regenerated and rejuvenated.

Before proceeding with the foot massage, a simple explanation for those who know nothing about reflexology reassures the recipient that this is a trustworthy, natural process that will encourage them to let go of unwanted issues and make them feel much better about who and what they are.

> *For healing to occur we need to work with, not against, the manifestation of illness, as it is an expression of all that is going on within.*

Relief of common ailments through the reflexology massage

Reflexology relieves common ailments through the subconscious release of emotional fears that traumatize the mind, distort the body and distress the soul. The relief of letting go eases all aspects of the whole and places the individual back on track for a more fulfilling, satisfying and creative reality.

Healing occurs more naturally when:

- the mind accepts and expresses its individuality
- personal talents are realized and utilized.
- there is pure love.

Recuperation occurs when there is:

- physical relief from distressing symptoms
- eradication of the upsetting emotion behind the dis-ease
- a change of mind to avoid re-occurrence
- inner harmony and peace
- an interest in getting better.

All this is facilitated and made possible through reflexology, which encourages individuals to help themselves to a better way of life.

> *Healing forces are within, not without …*
> *natural therapies merely facilitate the co-ordination of*
> *the mental and spiritual forces.*
> *The body can and does heal itself.*

04

preparing for the reflexology massage

In this chapter you will learn:
- to trust your intuition!

To begin!

Reflexology is incredibly easy to learn and apply since it is an inborn skill waiting to be alerted and utilized, it is like many instinctive acts that are frequently performed to relieve irritations and discomfort, such as:

- rubbing the skin to ease bumps or aching joints and muscles
- smearing saliva to soothe bites or stem minor blood flows
- scratching to relieve itching and irritability
- stroking, patting or hugging when upset or grieving
- massaging dull, numb areas to stimulate circulation.

This natural form of healing is instinctive knowledge best acquired when guided by intuition. The only pre-requisite is an appreciation of life and all it stands for, so that the potential for leading an outstanding existence can be realized.

Intent profoundly influences the outcome.

Reflexology is particularly beneficial when you are:

- stuck in a rut
- lacking direction
- feeling alone and misunderstood
- wondering what life is all about
- believing there is more to making a living
- questioning what the world is coming to.

With this natural form of healing everything is put into perspective and the mind shift that occurs makes the difference between 'having a life' and 'living life to the full'!

Ready to begin? Let's get started!

> *Only by venturing into the unknown do we appreciate the fullness and beauty of life.*

General preparation

The equipment required for reflexology consists mainly of standard household goods. Prepare these in advance to create a peaceful ambience to enhance the process.

- bed, settee, reclining chair or massage couch
- several pillows
- fresh, clean sheets in summer plus blankets, duvets or quilts in winter

- cushions, a stool or chair for the administrator
- a plastic bowl or foot bath
- recently laundered towels
- powder and/or aromatic oils or creams
- purified water and two glasses.

Optional extras include:

- an aroma lamp, aromatherapy oils (see Taking it Further, page 209)
- a music centre, ideally with a repeat button
- some soothing tapes or compact discs (see Taking it Further, page 211)
- an activated telephone answering machine or service to avoid interruption
- a 'Do not disturb' notice
- dimmer switch
- soft-coloured candles
- bird table
- fountain or running water
- Rescue Remedy (page 8)
- calcium tablets in case of cramp.

Carefully choose the furnishings.

- pastel colours sub-consciously soothe the senses
- bright colours stimulate and can heighten volatile feelings.

If possible, create as peaceful a setting as possible, in a subdued environment so that the recipient can escape the frenetic hustle and bustle of the outside world, and drift into a blissful state of relaxation. Remember, however, that once the eyes are closed, all external impressions are shut out and reflexology steps in and induces inner harmony.

> *Healing occurs when we go from a state of discomfort and distress, to one of harmony and ease.*

Preparation of the recipient

Before commencing a reflexology massage, briefly explain the following to the recipient, whether or not they have previously experienced this form of healing.

Step 1: explanation of reflexology
- what reflexology is (page 2)
- how it works (page 19–21)
- possible experiences before, during and after the massage (pages 44–8)
- the reasons for any reactions (pages 46–7)
- why it is advisable to drink plenty of purified water after the massage (page 47).

Those who are on prescribed medication should first advise their specialist of their intention to have reflexology so that appropriate adjustments can be made to the dosage, since there can be immediate improvements as the healing process becomes accelerated.

The reflexology massage is even more effective when administered one hour prior to the next dose of medication because this is the time when the influence of drugs is minimal and the body is in its most vulnerable and receptive state.

Once the formalities are over, invite the recipient to soak their bare feet in a foot spa or plastic bowl for a few minutes.

Step 2: the foot bath
- use warm water in winter and cool water in summer
- add a sprig or drop of lavender oil to enhance relaxation
- in summer, a drop of peppermint oil cools and refreshes
- provide a small clean towel to dry the feet.

This is an ideal time to chat, explain reflexology and find out more about the client. Then invite the recipient to lie as flat as possible on the bed, lazy-boy or couch, in a comfortable position.

Step 3: make the client comfortable
- place one pillow beneath the head, if required
- bolster the knees and lower legs with pillows to flatten and relax the spine
- cover with a light sheet in summer and a warm blanket or duvet in winter for modesty and also to retain heat lost through relaxation
- sit comfortably at the recipient's feet, with the recipient's feet at an appropriate height for massage
- invite the recipient to close their eyes
- prepare yourself (pages 34–5) and the recipient by taking in three long, deep breaths, having explained the breathing process beforehand

- shake powder into one hand, rub the hands together and then with both hands spread it gently over the feet and between the toes. This not only facilitates the massage but also makes the recipient less self-conscious, especially when there is an unpleasant odour from extreme anxiety
- discourage conversation during the massage to allow the recipient to drift into the tranquil alpha state and reconnect with the inner self.
- it is now time for the warm-up technique (pages 56–63).

Treat everybody as the most important person in the world.

Personal preparation

Although it is extremely rewarding to see amazing results so quickly, it is important to remember that the administrator is only the conduit or facilitator, who directs universal energies towards the recipient encouraging them to generate their own healing from within. For the most beneficial massage:

Step 1: Create trust
- gently rest the recipient's feet in the palms of both hands, in a comfortable position (Figure 7).

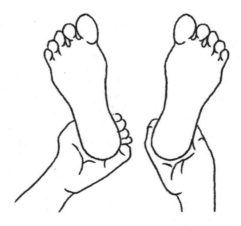

figure 7 resting the feet in both hands

Step 2: breathe and relax

- invite the recipient to join you in closing the eyes and taking three long, deep breaths, holding each breath for as long as possible
- as you breathe, consciously relax particularly tense areas, especially in the
  - neck
  - shoulders
  - back
  - upper arms
- concentrate on taut parts in your own body and breathe into them
- then breathe naturally
- with the eyes still closed, centre and focus inwards, directing energies towards your heart
- clear your mind
- use your hands to tune into the recipient's energies and access what they are truly feeling through what the feet are 'saying'
- forget about trying to please and just be yourself
- make up your mind to enjoy every second of the session
- be prepared to vary the pressure of the massage movements from being gentle but firm, for physical ease, to barely touching the skin's surface for personal enlightenment, in order to satisfy the needs of mind, body and soul
- for particularly sensitive souls, visualize two beautiful pink bubbles around you and the recipient so that each of you can enjoy your individual energy and space
- allow yourself to be intuitively guided.

During and after the reflexology massage, both you and the recipient should experience complete serenity, inner peace and a tremendous boost of life-force energy.

> We have all brought a special gift to the planet ... ourselves and our own individual uniqueness.

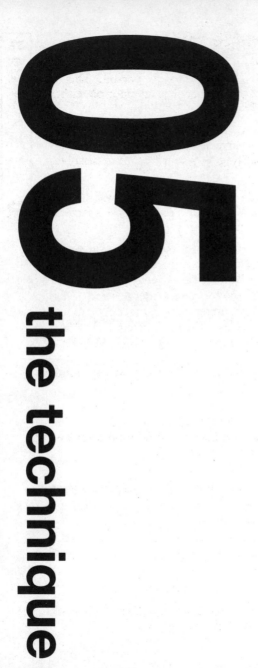

05

the technique

In this chapter you will know:
- to tune into the true essence of life and be guided every step of the way.

Reflexology massage movements

An effective reflexology massage relies primarily on the thera-peutic touch, which differs from person to person. This is important since any caress of the skin evokes an emotion, either consciously or subconsciously.

Aggressive, threatening actions make one recoil or lash out in self-defence, whereas acts of love and acceptance boost self-confidence and create a trusting environment that dissolves distress and dis-ease.

Reflexology values a sensitive application with pure intent. Complete acceptance is essential since the administrator's feelings are immediately conveyed to the recipient.

The massage movements gently loosen and break down the fixation with time and release mind, body and soul from being entrapped by belief systems that no longer apply, so that they no longer interfere with personal growth and development.

The therapeutic movements of the reflexology massage:

- naturalize all bodily functions
- calm the nerves
- soothe over-sensitivity or increase sensitivity when numb with fear
- create inner harmony
- stimulate the circulatory and lymphatic systems
- reduce high blood pressure and increase low blood pressure
- ease aches and pains
- strengthen the immune system
- pacify over-active and stimulate under-active glands and organs
- arouse sluggish bodily parts
- relax muscles
- relieve tension and distress
- reduce swelling
- eliminate toxic substances
- energize and rejuvenate mind, body and soul.

The need for touch increases during times of illness, distress or insecurity. The therapeutic touch of massage can:

- pacify
- induce confidence
- reassure

- free from distress
- create trust
- increase acceptability.

Until recently the reflexology technique concentrated on the all-important physical and mechanical approach, but with the rapid shift in consciousness, it has expanded to keep abreast of modern needs, which makes it one of the most all-encompassing therapies.

Tuning into the recipient's requirements assists in determining the type of touch required, whether it should be firm or light. Physical people tend to prefer a harder approach initially, but this modifies as personal awareness increases. Spiritual souls generally favour a gentler, non-physical approach, but there may be times when they need to be brought down to earth and grounded with a slightly firmer touch.

Four simple movements assist in meeting the ever-changing personal needs of the individual and these can be personalized through an adjustment of pressure. These variations can differ from one part of the foot to another and from treatment to treatment, depending on the fluctuating physical and emotional requirements of the recipient.

The four reflexology techniques
- rotation technique
- caterpillar movement
- stroking or milking (2 types)
- feather-stroke or healing.

Knowing the amount of pressure required is an intuitive process. It can vary considerably from one extreme to the other, from being really firm in one massage to having no physical contact at all during another.

The four techniques are now explained in detail. Practise them on the hand first, to gain confidence.

Technique 1: rotation technique

- gently rest the tip of the appropriate digit on the reflex
- apply slight pressure and hold for a while

- slowly release to activate the energy channels
- a tingling sensation may be felt
- without moving the digit, create a vibration by gently gyrating the digit on the point of contact
- if resistance is felt or the reflex feels drained of energy, lightly press onto the reflexes and hold the pressure momentarily
- very slowly ease off
- lightly rest the digits on the skin for a while before moving onto subsequent reflexes (Figure 8).

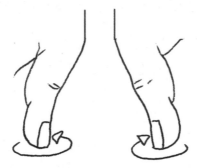

figure 8 rotation technique

Effects of the rotation technique
- opens energy channels
- raises consciousness
- soothes nerves
- balances and harmonizes.

Technique 2: caterpillar movement

- place the tip of both thumbs lightly on the skin's surface, one on each corresponding foot
- gently drop the thumbs so that their pads rest lightly on the skin
- rock the thumbs back onto their tips and, in so doing, move them forwards a fraction
- ease the thumbs once again back down onto their pads
- continue to 'walk' the thumbs forward in this manner (Figure 9).

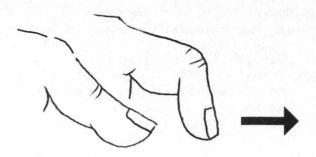

figure 9 caterpillar movement

Effects of the caterpillar movement
- relaxes muscular tension
- eases physical distress
- relieves aches and pains
- adjusts mental activity.

Technique 3: stroking or milking

Method 1
- apply after the rotation and caterpillar movements
- place the thumbs or fingers firmly but lightly on the reflexes
- reassuringly stroke the skin's surface in long soothing sweeps or shorter strokes along the reflexes whilst applying slight pressure (Figure 10).

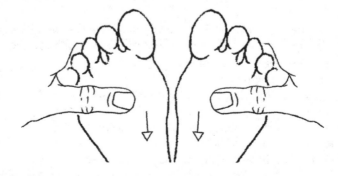

figure 10 stroking or milking method 1

Method 2

- stroke thumb over thumb or finger over finger (Figure 11).

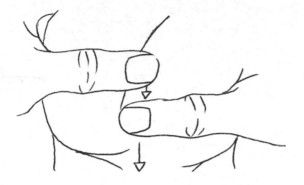

figure 11 stroking or milking method 2

Effects of the stroking or milking methods
- soothes disturbed emotions
- creates inner harmony
- eliminates disruptive feelings
- boosts self-confidence.

Technique 4: feather-stroke or healing procedure

- apply at the end of each sequence of movements on every reflex
- stroke the skin's surface very lightly or caress the energies just above the skin in the auric space by alternating the digits (Figure 12).

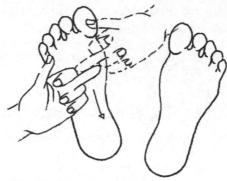

figure 12 feather-stroke or healing procedure

Effects of the feather-stroke or healing procedure
- reconnects with soul purpose
- accentuates the inner essence
- re-establishes contact with the true self.

---

*Our souls came to earth for
the richest experience – not the poorest,
for the most – not the least*

Healing hands

The effectiveness of the reflexology massage lies in the utilization of the fingers and thumbs and the manner in which they embrace the feet. Furthermore the use of all digits greatly enhances the healing process since each has a unique energy and different vibration and effect.

Effective use of digits

- **thumbs** raise consciousness and improve mental activity by creating a much-needed balance between the intellect and intuition
- **second fingers** reconnect individuals with their innermost feelings whilst also soothing, pacifying and making space just to be and believe in oneself
- **middle fingers** stimulate and activate to ensure that extraordinary ideas become a worthwhile reality

- **ring fingers** generate new concepts for greater understanding and enhanced co-operation
- **the little fingers** encourage expansion beyond the tried and tested, as well as the courage to venture and explore the unknown.

The effects of the massage movements

For best results, massage every reflex in both feet with each of the aforementioned movements, giving the greatest attention to the brain, spinal, solar plexus and endocrine gland reflexes. One and a half to two hours may be required initially to complete a full massage but, with confidence and practice, this can be reduced to an hour or fractionally less.

Each movement during the reflexology massage either:

- activates by toning and strengthening sluggish, hypo-active, dull areas that require stimulation, or
- pacifies by calming and soothing nervous, hyperactive or tense areas that need to let go.

Whether giving reflexology to maintain health or to relieve specific symptoms and ease dis-ease, always massage both feet thoroughly, concentrating on congested, swollen areas or parts that lack vibrancy. These are easily detected on the skin's surface in the following ways:

- a resistance or hardness is detected due to fear, anxiety or vulnerability
- there is an intense drawing of energy due to the need for increased vitality and rejuvenation
- flatness, unresponsiveness or dullness from feeling drained and exhausted is evident.

On these unnatural reflexes either:

- lightly rest the most appropriate digit onto the affected spot to re-energize
- then apply gentle pressure
- finally slowly release until there is minimal contact and a gush of energy.

or

- increase the rotation technique to reawaken and stimulate the reflex.

Respecting personal belief systems makes it intuitively easier to know which is best for the individual. Although results may be amazing, even after one treatment, by not taking credit for the healing there is less likelihood of a loss of confidence when there is, from time to time, no apparent reaction. The outcome of treatments may be affected by the recipient's choice to improve or otherwise. This is more likely when the recipient receives greater sympathy and attention during illness than when they are well and so they subconsciously block or slow down the healing because it is not in their interest to get better. It can also occur when, at a deep subconscious level, an individual feels incapable of meeting other people's expectations and so chooses to remain incapacitated.

When the administrator consciously puts their personal will to one side and allows instinct to step in, the most favourable outcome is ensured.

> *The best way of doing anything has never been found.*

Sensations experienced during the reflexology massage

The recipient drifts into the exquisite alpha level of consciousness during reflexology massage. In this state there is an acute awareness of surrounding noise and activity but any concern is overridden by a pleasant detachment that dispenses with the need to be involved. In this way, the recipient never loses conscious control, despite appearing to be in a deep sleep.

A variety of very individual sensations are experienced during a reflexology massage. It is impossible to determine how a recipient is likely to react.

- extreme tenderness indicates a high level of tension and anxiety
- excessive sensitivity acts as an alarm that alerts the whole to be defensive due to nervousness, fear or insecurity.

Knowing what possible reactions can occur puts the recipient's mind at rest and allows them to fully appreciate the process of letting go with ease. Here are some of the responses that may be experienced:

- heat loss as the body relaxes and lets off steam
- a sinking feeling as the mind and body relax

- a floating sensation as burdens dissipate taking a weight off the whole
- twitching and jerking due to previously deprived, tense areas receiving a sudden surge of vitality
- plucking hand movements from the frustration of having to deal with uncertain situations
- 'pins and needles' or numbness in the hands from the subconscious dread or thwarting of handling certain circumstances
- snoring to release deeply suppressed emotions that have been kept close to the chest
- the appearance of beautiful colours, ranging from subdued, subtle hues to exceptionally bright tints, even with the eyes closed.

Less common reactions include:

- out of body experiences as the soul temporarily leaves the body for a different point of view
- recall of previous life situations
- feeling a murky lining of emotional trash being pulled out of the body like a piece of material so that it can be finally dispensed with
- singing out loud songs such as 'Please release me'.

Bear in mind that whatever happens, no matter how peculiar or unexpected, is ideal for the individual concerned.

During reflexology massage, breathing becomes shallow and, at times, almost undetectable as the recipient drifts into other dimensions. For this reason, it is helpful to ask the recipient to take three deep breaths at the end of the session to bring themselves out of this incredibly relaxed state! There may be an initial reluctance to leave such a blissful state, so allow time.

Even greater benefit can be derived if the recipient is in bed and can roll over to sleep because they can then emerge in their own time feeling really fantastic!

Healing naturally occurs when there is a shift from a state of discomfort and distress, to one of harmony and ease.

After-effects of reflexology

It is important to explain to the recipient, the reasons for possible reactions so that they are aware of what to expect and why. As a revitalizing and rejuvenating therapy, the most common reaction to reflexology is renewed enthusiasm and vitality for life.

Some of the enjoyable after-effects

- clarity of thought
- increased tolerance
- improved concentration
- internal and external harmony
- greater confidence
- activities become more worthwhile
- abundant energy
- refreshing, deep sleep
- meaningful dreams
- greater awareness of body and soul needs
- more respect for mind, body and soul
- clearer direction
- deeper understanding of one's soul purpose
- improved quality of life.

It is also possible for there to be a complete personality change from being a disgruntled, aggressive, obstinate grouch, to being an affable, patient and accommodating soul.

Reflexology works with, and not against, the manifestations of illness to complete the cycle of dis-ease. It relies on the purification of mind, body and soul, which is only possible when old outdated belief systems and detrimental habits are eliminated, making way for a fresh start and a more meaningful approach to life.

Although the effects of this clearing process may initially be disturbing, exhausting or disruptive, once complete, there is a fantastic feeling of liberation and release. Any of the following are excellent signs that the body is helping itself to better health.

- a headache as past hurts come to a head for final eradication
- high temperatures to let off steam and eliminate heated emotions
- increased perspiration, which flushes out old fears
- runny eyes to unleash unshed tears and wash away hurtful sights
- a cold, or runny nose, which clears out past irritations
- skin rashes or eruptions as irrational, boiling emotions that get under the skin come to the surface and escape
- females may experience a more virulent vaginal discharge as frustrating female issues are eliminated
- increased urination that relieves one of wasteful emotions
- frequent, easier defecation to eliminate the wasteful remnants of life's processes
- temporary diarrhoea, as unnecessary nonsense and unreasonable pressure are dispensed with
- vivid recall of dreams to help comprehend life's on-going events.

Encourage the recipient to drink plenty of purified water after a reflexology massage to assist the flushing-through process and hasten the release of inhibiting thoughts and emotions that otherwise make life heavy going.

Life can be understood backwards but must be lived forwards!

Unusual but possible reactions

Natural stimulants evoke natural responses, so it is impossible to cause harm with the light, but firm, movements used in reflexology.

However, individuals continually challenge themselves to test their inner strength and resourcefulness in dealing with unexpected and apparently adverse situations as part of their growth experience. If a perceivably alarming reaction does occur during the reflexology session remain calm and be intuitively guided to know what steps to take.

As a non-invasive, natural therapy, reflexology can only cause dormant conditions to surface. If rapid, it may be disturbing and appear to be an adverse reaction – it is, in fact, an excellent sign that the healing process has been activated.

Palpitations, hyperventilation or panic can occur from the subconscious arousal of heart-wrenching emotions that require immediate release. Stay calm! Whenever a response causes concern, pacify by:

- immediately placing the digits on the solar plexus reflexes (pages 130–1)
- asking the recipient to take long, deep breaths and relax
- reassure the recipient that the reaction is temporary
- if available, administer Rescue Remedy to induce inner calm.

The recipient should begin to feel more tranquil almost immediately, but be patient if it takes a while.

Once the recipient has settled down take some soothing breaths and continue the massage. On completion encourage them to drink more purified water than usual to flush out any extra toxins. Also suggest that they return as soon as possible for further massage to continue balancing out the whole.

The above reactions are not common, but it is important to be aware of them so that appropriate action can be taken if necessary.

> *Everybody is completely responsible for their own thoughts, actions and reactions.*

First-aid reflexology

Ideally a complete massage on both feet is required for complete homoeostatis of mind, body and soul. Occasionally, however, insufficient time will dictate a 'quick massage', which is better than nothing. This entails:

- massaging all toes thoroughly (pages 76–98)
- soothing the spinal reflexes (pages 94–5)
- pacifying the solar plexus reflexes (pages 130–1)
- balancing the energy centres (page 128)
- always finishing with an overall massage of both feet (page 202).

To ease extreme discomfort in a particular part of the body:

- massage the distressed reflex(es) (see index, page 137)
- then calm the solar plexus reflexes (pages 130–1)
- continue with the natural procedure or the 'quick massage' above.

Rule of thumb

For any disorder, a complete reflexology massage is required with emphasis on:

- the nervous system and solar plexus reflexes to calm the mind and relieve pain, fear and anxiety
- the endocrine gland reflexes to soothe disturbed emotions and create inner harmony
- the affected gland or organ reflexes to relax the distressed area and ease the symptoms of dis-ease.

> *Knowledge is attained through positive and negative actions and reactions, with health being the neutral position of life.*

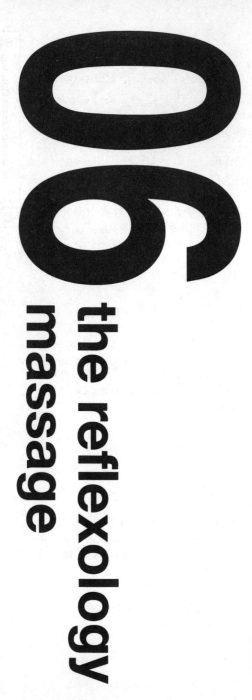

06

the reflexology massage

In this chapter you will realize:
• that when we understand that everything is cyclical then the massaging process is a pleasure.

The sequence

Always begin the reflexology massage with a general massage, which is known as the warm-up (pages 56–63). The caressing movements of the warm up:

- encourage initial relaxation
- create a trusting relationship
- provide an ideal opportunity to gauge recipient's needs through feeling the feet.

The order of the reflexology massage is then as follows:

Step 1: massage the brain and sensory reflexes
The central nervous system is mainly reflected in the toes (page 76), where the brain and major sensory reflexes are situated. Massage of this area:

- calms or stimulates the mind
- soothes or excites the emotions
- pacifies or heightens the senses.

Step 2: massage of the spinal and solar plexus reflexes
The spine (pages 94–5), reflected onto the knobbly ridges of bone along the inside edges of both feet, and the solar plexus reflexes (pages 130–1) is situated in the hollows beneath the balls of the feet. Massage of this area:

- pacifies or excites the nerves
- relaxes or strengthens the musculature
- releases overall tension
- improves circulation
- enhances the natural functioning of all bodily systems.

Step 3: massage the reflexes of the neck and throat
The lymphatic system, which infiltrates the whole body, yet is especially evident in the neck and throat (page 110), is reflected in the toe necks. Massage of this area:

- relieves neck and throat tension
- facilitates the exchange of natural life-forces, e.g. air
- opens the avenues of expression, e.g. speech
- assists in the intake of energizing forces, e.g. food.

Step 4: massage the endocrine gland reflexes

The endocrine system's reflexes are situated throughout both feet. Massaging these reflexes:

• balances and harmonizes mind, body and soul.

Step 5: massage the reflexes of the upper torso

The reflexes of the respiratory and cardiac systems, the chest, heart, breasts, upper arms and upper back are located on the balls of both feet (pages 113–135). Massaging these reflexes:

• boosts self-esteem and self-worth
• provides space for self-expression
• releases retained emotions from the chest
• eases snoring
• soothes respiratory tension
• stabilizes the heart
• regulates the blood flow.

Step 6: massage the abdominal reflexes

The bulk of the digestive system, part of the urinary tract, reproductive and excretory systems are reflected in the insteps (pages 137–179). Massaging these reflexes:

• harmonizes the digestive process
• assists in the effective utilization of nutrients
• eases the assimilation and absorption of life processes
• nourishes mind, body and soul
• forms and maintains fulfilling relationships
• relieves abdominal discomfort
• re-energizes and rejuvenates.

Step 7: massage the lower torso reflexes

The skeletal and muscular, as well as the main parts of the excretory and reproductive systems are located in the heels, (pages 181–196), which reflects all the pelvic contents. Massaging these reflexes:

• revitalizes mind, body and soul with renewed energy
• enthuses the whole for lively participation on the journey through life
• enhances personal growth and development
• increases individual security
• relieves muscular and skeletal tension.

Step 7: the finale

The finale (pages 198–208) ends the reflexology massage sequence.

The invigorating massage and manipulation of both feet:

- releases any remaining tension
- loosens the tight grip on life
- enhances relaxation, whilst stimulating mind, body and soul
- increases flexibility for overall well-being.

> *The cycles of nature defy a linear approach to life.*

General observations of the feet

In their natural state feet are vibrant and pliant making it easy for them to adapt and fit into the ever-changing events of life's circumstance.

When alarmed, they become tense and increasingly rigid with a build-up of resistance that temporarily hampers progress. When the going gets really tough, the skin on the feet is more likely to harden and thicken in areas of perceived vulnerability, either to protect or to conceal true emotions. The actual position of calluses, corns and extra skin makes it possible to pinpoint areas of subconscious issues that manifest in the tissues.

The natural texture of the skin should be firm but supple to display the inner effervescence and high energy levels. Look for the following skin characteristics:

- flaccidity due to
  - giving in too easily under pressure
  - a temporary lack of inner strength and substance

- toughness from
  - perceived difficulty in making personal progress
  - creating a barrier against being hurt
  - acting in defiance

- shiny and/or blistered as a result of
  - continual friction that rubs one up the wrong way

- flaky due to
  - irritabilities that get under the skin
  - a 'flaky' approach to life

- peeling indicating
  - a period of transition
  - letting go of the old and making way for the new.

Feet are naturally flesh coloured and can comfortably blend into the changing hues of on-going circumstances that colour the journey through life. Alterations in skin colouration highlight fluctuations in dominant moods and overriding feelings that come to the surface from time to time. Several different colours can be present on the feet at any one time and these can perpetually alter with shifting emotions. Significant colours include:

- white from being
  - drained
  - tired
  - exhausted
  - divinely guided
  - enlightened

- red due to
  - heated emotions
  - intense anger
  - extreme frustration
  - embarrassment
  - passion

- brown from being
  - 'browned off'
  - down to earth
  - in touch with nature

- yellow due to
  - exceptional annoyance
  - a jaundiced outlook
  - overwhelming enthusiasm

- green from
  - tinges of envy
  - enjoying one's space

- black and blue arising from
  - feeling emotionally battered, with the depth of colour, indicating the degree of hurt
  - bruised sentiment

- being momentarily in the dark
- needing an expressive outlet

- orange, a mixture of red and yellow, is likely to indicate
  - being 'pissed off' at being continually upset
  - eagerly wishing to communicate one's brilliant ideas.

Energies, absorbed from the sun and earth, are channelled through the body differently to provide a more balanced approach and prospective of life. The reason for each soul setting foot on earth can, in this way, be more deeply understood. Reflections on the right and left feet are as follows:

- the right foot reflects the right side of the body, conveying the more positive, masculine energies, which carry the markings of past experiences
- the left foot represents the left side of the body, giving preference to the negative female energies and is far more impressed by present thoughts and feelings
- every cell, however, contains both male/female, as well as positive/negative, energies to varying degrees according to current thoughts, feelings, actions and reactions.

The angle of the feet signifies an individual's perceived position in life whilst walking, standing, sitting and lying.

Differing angles of feet

- when walking feet indicate the direction in which one is headed
  - parallel feet naturally show that the individual is on track with their soul journey
  - open feet are too accommodating and continually try to please, which can throw them off track
  - pigeon-toed feet temporarily lack confidence and subconsciously cut themselves off from the outside world to soul search

- when standing, the space between the feet shows the openness of the mind and the scan of personal interest
  - together the feet stand to attention on their best behaviour or are completely focused on the task in hand
  - open feet open-mindedly embrace all that comes between them
  - inverted feet reveal self-centredness or uncertainty

- when sitting the toes point in the direction of interest or indicate an overriding thought that holds the greatest attention
- when lying in a prone position the feet should be supply upright
  - if drawn to the right they show that the mind is dealing with past issues
  - if leaning towards the left side of the body the individual is forward planning and projecting the mind into the future.

The characteristics of our feet reveal the story of our life.

The warm-up: general loosening-up techniques for initial relaxation

The caressing movements of the warm up:

- create a trusting relationship
- provide an ideal opportunity to gauge recipient needs.

Adapt the following techniques to suit recipient's needs:

Step 1: caressing the feet top and bottom

- gently stroke the top of the right foot, hand over hand, towards yourself (Figure 13)
- then stroke the sole of the right foot with the backs of the hands (Figure 14)
- repeat on the left foot.

The Language of the Feet, also written by Chris Stormer and published by Hodder and Stoughton, provides deeper insight into the ever-changing and fascinating characteristics of the feet. With life constantly changing, and people striving to progress, this understanding makes it easier to tune into the recipient's individual needs, which differ from massage to massage!

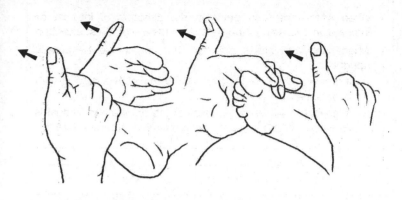

figure 13 caressing the tops

> *To reacquaint the souls and create a trusting relationship.*

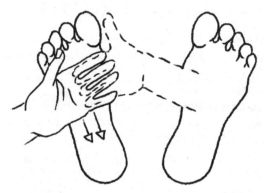

figure 14 stroking the soles

Step 2: exploratory and releasing massage

- place all fingertips on top of the toes, on the right foot
- with tiny circular movements and a gentle pushing, kneading movement, massage, with all fingers, from the toes up to the ankle
- separate the hands at the ankle and continue to massage either side of the right ankle thoroughly (Figure 16)
- repeat on the left foot.

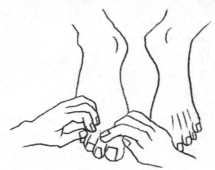

figure 15 massaging one foot at a time

Exploratory and releasing massage locates and eases back tension arising from issues:

- that have been placed in the background, or
- that one has turned one's back on, or
- are perceived to be going on behind one's back.

Step 3: massaging the ankle

- place your left fingers on the outside of the recipient's right ankle-bone and your right fingers on the inside ankle-bone
- initially simultaneously massage around the right ankle bone, with fairly firm, definite circular movements (Figure 16)
- ease off the pressure until there is little or no contact, whilst at the same time reducing the number of fingers until only the middle fingers remain massaging lightly
- repeat on the left foot, adjusting the role of the hands.

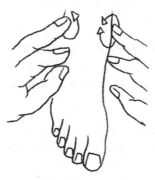

figure 16 massaging the ankles

Massaging the ankles:

- loosens the hip-bones
- reassures the individual
- encourages them to believe in themselves.

Step 4: foot shake

- place the mounds at the bases of your thumbs in the hollows either side of the right ankle-bones so that they rest comfortably
- keeping contact at all times, move one hand up and the other hand down to coax the whole of the right foot to swing from side to side (Figure 17)
- with practice this movement can be speeded up or slowed down as required
- repeat on the left foot, changing the role of the hands.

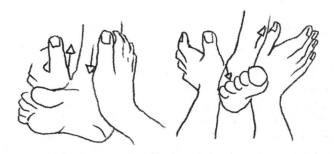

figure 17 foot shake

Shaking the foot:

- loosens tension in adapting to life's ups and downs
- increases flexibility in one's approach to relationships
- eases the strain of holding or being held back
- provides the confidence to step out and move ahead.

Step 5: the Achilles pull

- for this next movement the recipient must be lying flat
- rest their right heel in the palm of your left hand and align your right hand on top of the same foot (Figure 18)
- gently but firmly extend their right heel towards yourself, stretching the right leg, until a slight resistance is felt

- repeat about 3 times before going onto the left foot and swapping the role of the hands.

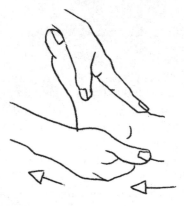

figure 18 Achilles pull

Pulling the Achilles:

- opens energy pathways
- elongates and realigns the spine
- releases pressure on entrapped, impinged nerves
- eases neck and head tension.

Step 6 : Achilles stretch

- once again rest the right heel in the palm of your left hand and align your right hand on top of the same foot
- this time use the upper hand to gently, but firmly bend the foot downwards
- extend the upper surface of the foot as far as possible without resistance
- repeat about 3 times
- repeat on the left foot, reversing the role of the hands
- this movement can be alternated with the Achilles pull.

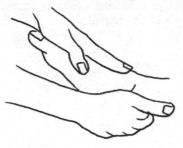

figure 19 Achilles stretch

Stretching the Achilles:

- creates greater awareness of when to hold back and when to step forward
- makes one more open being stretched from time to time.

Step 7: knuckle down massage

- gently support the right toes with your left hand
- make a fist with your right hand
- place the flat surface between the knuckles below the toe necks towards the outer edge of the sole of the right foot
- sensitively stroke the soles from top to bottom
- massage in strips from the outer to the inner edges of the foot (Figure 20)
- repeat on the left foot, reversing the role of the hands.

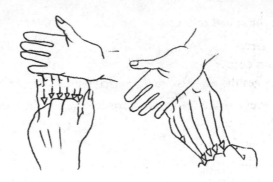

figure 20 knuckle down massage

A knuckle down massage:

- encourages one to 'knuckle in' and deal with the tasks in hand
- assists in confronting all that comes one's way
- opens the energy pathways
- clears the way for ideas to be put into practice.

Step 8: spinal reflex rub

- use the heel of the right palm to stroke the inside arch of the right instep, towards the recipient
- apply slight pressure to the bony ridge on the way up
- gently drag the heel of the hand back to the big toe
- massage in this way a few times
- then repeat on the left arch with the heel of the left palm.

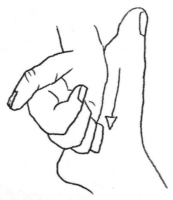

figure 21 spinal reflex rub

Rubbing the spinal reflexes:

- calms nerves
- appeases core issues
- encourages the alpha state of consciousness.

Between every sequence stroke both feet, from the toes to the ankles, to:

- create overall harmony
- enhance the effects of the procedure
- accelerate the healing process
- reassure the recipient.

> *Live well for today*
> *For yesterday is but a dream*
> *And tomorrow a vision,*
> *But today well lived*
> *Makes every yesterday*
> *A dream of happiness*
> *And every tomorrow*
> *A vision of hope.*

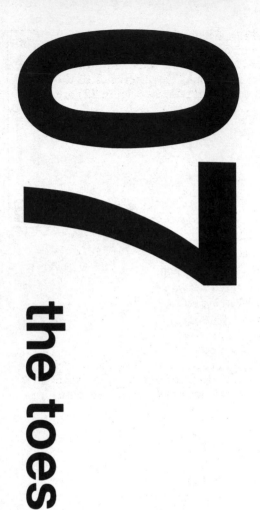

07

the toes

All the toes reflect the head, which, through the brain, consciously, subconsciously and unconsciously, determines the condition and health of mind, body and soul. All this is accurately reflected through the state and characteristics of the feet. For this reason the head and brain reflexes (Figure 22) are always massaged first.

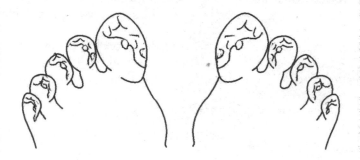

figure 22 brain reflexes on all toes

The spinal cord reflexes are then massaged because the nerve fibres infiltrate the whole body. Reflexology ensures that messages to and from the brain are accurately conveyed with ease (Figure 22).

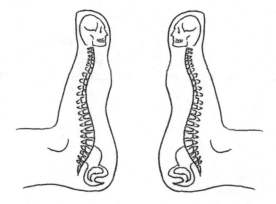

figure 23 spinal cord and vertebral reflexes

Life is an adventure of the mind, that makes the impossible possible.

Toe reflexes

Each toe reflects half the head and face. The right toes mirror the right side of the head, revealing the effect of past thoughts and memories, whilst the left toes reflect the left side of the head to show present ways of thinking and current ideas.

- the toe pads mirror the face, with the right side of the face on the right toe pads, and the left side of the face on the left toe pads
- the outer edges (on the little toe sides) portray the sides of the head
- the inner edges (on the big toe sides) represent the meeting of the two sides of the head and the core of one's being
- the upper surfaces of the toes reflect the back of the head and neck
- the toe nails represent the cranium.

Each set of toes reflects different aspect of the thinking process (Figure 24) as follows:

- the big toes are the thinking toes that reflect intellectual, intuitive and spiritual choices
- the second toes, known as the feeling toes, show personal thoughts regarding past feelings (right toes) and current emotions (left toes)
- the third toes, the doing toes, reveal ideas of what could have been done or not done (right toes) and currently what to do or not do (left toes)
- the fourth toes, the communication toes, mirror concepts regarding previous relationships (right toes) and ways in which to communicate in the present (left toes)
- the little toes, the security/family toes, reproduce the impact of past social beliefs (right toes) and present personal values (left toes).

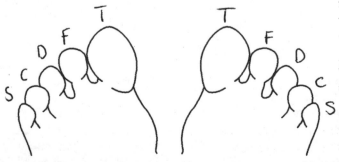

figure 24 specific toe meanings

Key

T = thinking toes
F = feeling toes
D = doing toes
C = communication toes
S = security/family toes

The head reflexes, on each pair of toes pads, can also be divided into six horizontal sections (Figure 25) for greater insight into how individuals think and face up to their reality. These are as follows:

- the first uppermost sections reflect the brain, hair and sinuses (thoughts)
- the second strips contain the forehead and midbrain reflexes (expression of thoughts)
- the third upper central mounds reflect the eyes and pineal gland (feelings)
- the fourth lower central mounds mirror the nose, pituitary gland, cheek and ears (doing, actions and reactions)
- the fifth zone portrays the mouth, teeth and gum (communications and relationships)
- the lower edges denote the jaw reflexes (basic security).

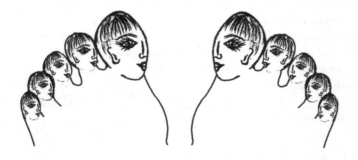

figure 25 face reflexes on all toes

Key

T = thoughts
F = feelings
D = doing, actions and reactions
C = communication
S = security, stability, mobility

Natural characteristics of toes

Healthy toes:

- stand supply upright
- are pliant, yet firm and flexible
- have well shaped firm pads
- emit a vibrant fleshy hue.

Impact of tension on the toes

Social constraints and limited belief systems place physical restraints on the mind, causing the muscles to contract, which puts pressure on the brain. This can also substantially reduce the size of the cranium, which physiologically deprives the brain cells of essential life-forces and denies them the opportunity to function to their maximum potential. The following symptoms may possibly occur:

- fear of expressing one's own unique concepts
- lack of concentration
- disturbed thought processes
- irritability
- impatience
- headaches or migraines
- pressure on the mind
- no space to think
- baldness as hair follicles become trapped
- throwing fits
- aggravated senses
- distorted, amplified, exaggerated and/or misconstrued perceptions.

Altered state of toes

Thought patterns have a direct impact on the stature, shape, size and skin of the toes, which, under distressing circumstances, can noticeably change their natural characteristics.

Stature of toes

The stature of toes reveals the degree of confidence in standing up and facing the world with personal concepts and ideals.

Unnatural toe statures

Rigidity reflects uncertainty and insecurity because of:

- set beliefs
- unbending attitude
- an obdurate approach to life.

Toes that lean forwards, over the soles:

- desperately try to get their point of view across
- wish to be 'in your face'
- stick out their necks.

Those that pull backwards and upwards:

- keep their opinions to themselves
- push their own ideas into the background
- shy away from having to share their true thoughts
- try to avoid confrontation.

Toes that turn to the left indicate:

- that the mind is being projected into the future
- forward planning.

Toes that turn to the right:

- look back for old ideas
- hang on to outdated beliefs
- are reliving the past.

Bent toes:

- bow when succumbing to other belief systems
- do not stand up to face the world with their own personal concepts
- charge ahead without thinking
- go head first into life regardless of the consequences.

Shape of toes

The shape of the toes reveals how ideas take shape, which influences the shape of things to come.

Altered shapes of toes

- misshapen toes are contorted from trying to adjust and fit into alien belief patterns that do not suit them
- boxed toes contain or box in their own ideas for fear of the consequences
- pointed toes go straight to the point usually with sharp, witty or hurtful comments
- squashed toes have quelled their ideas and deprived themselves of the opportunity to bring their bright ideas out into the open
- dented toes knock their own way of thinking believing them to be inadequate or ridiculous in the eyes of others.

Size of toes

The size of the toes reveals an individual's capacity to think.

Different sized toes

Toes shrink when there is perceived to be:

- little or no opportunity to think for oneself
- when there is a deep fear of what others may think.

Toes expand and can become overly large when:

- bursting with brilliant notions but have no perceivable outlet
- keeping one's own ideas contained
- full of nonsense.

Condition of the skin on the toes

The condition of the skin on the toes reveals the effect of conditioned belief systems and the state of mind that one is in.

Unnatural skin conditions

Hard skin arises from:

- difficulty in thinking in the same way as others
- covering up or protecting unique concepts
- concealing one's true identity.

Blistered skin occurs when there is:

- friction
- a conflict of ideas.

Flaking skin arises out of:

- irritability
- a 'flaky' approach to life.

Peeling skin is:

- evidence of old beliefs being released to make way for new thoughts.

Shiny skin indicates an innate desire:

- to expose one's personal notions but meeting resistance
- have light thrown on a situation
- conflicting beliefs.

Weeping skin occurs when there is:

- deep anxiety
- extreme unhappiness
- fear of implementing one's own unusual concepts
- terror about what others think.

Colour of toes

The colouring of the skin on the toes reveals the emotional aspect of either caring or inconsiderate thought patterns that charge or drain energies from the specific chakra centres.

Colourful changes

White toes signify:

- exhaustion
- too drained to think
- enlightenment
- spirituality.

Black or blue toes indicate

- hurt notions
- the need for clarity to think

Green toes reveal:

- envy
- feeling sick at the thought
- loving opinions.

Yellow toes occur when:

- fed up
- delighted with specific types of mental activity.

Orange toes are indicative of:

- mixed views
- an annoyance
- joyous glee at the very thought of something.

Red toes highlight:

- extreme frustration
- infuriation
- embarrassing thoughts.

NB More than one colour can appear on the toes, in which case use the head and toe divisions (pages 24 and 25) to derive even greater understanding.

Nervous dis-orders

The state of the mind arises from the content or discontent of the soul and affects the content or discontent of the body.

Dis-ease is the outward manifestation of internal uneasiness, unhappiness and tension, which can really 'get on the nerves'. A variety of specific symptoms reveal particular thought patterns, which, when run through the body jog stored memories and can upset the emotional balance, causing further internal havoc and physical unrest. This leads to a belief of:

- being out of control
- being pressurized

- feeling anxious
- not being able to cope.

All of these can tip the balance either way in an attempt to either:

- overcompensate and get on top of the situation, or
- give in.

Consequently, one or more may occur:

	Too much	Too little
Irritability	sets the 'nerves on edge'	numbness or paralysis from 'deadening the nerves'
Tolerance	dis-ease to please causing antagonism and ill-feelings	complete intolerance manifesting in allergic reaction
Patience	endurance and persistence that test the patience	impatience leading to edginess and irritation
Sensitivity	increased concern, too much involvement and a tendency to overreact and take umbrage	indifference, unresponsiveness, coldness or unconcern

When under strain, the nervous impulses, which are conveyed along finely tuned, highly sensitive nerve fibres, become distorted or traumatized by threatening thought patterns. This can lead to one or more of the following signs:

- pain as an outward display of deep emotional hurt
- aching from an intense longing for love and recognition
- tension due to extreme anxiety, frustration, fear or concern
- nervousness from on-going uncertainty and inner havoc
- infections, inflammations and high temperatures as festering thoughts become unleashed
- convulsions erupting from fits of rage that distort the brain waves and throw brain activity off course.

Nervous dis-orders relieved by reflexology

The following are ways in which reflexology effectively relieves specific nervous ailments:

- aches: replaces the aching need for recognition through the touch of acceptance.
- acne: dissipates unexpressed frustration and anger at the insecurity of facing the world with one's personal concepts and ideas by encouraging belief in oneself
- addictions: replaces the need to escape perceived pressures by creating greater inner understanding
- adenoids: overcomes feelings of inadequacy through recognition of one's capabilities
- aging: eases personal concerns and apprehension and constantly rejuvenates mind, body and soul
- Alzheimer's disease: dismisses the belief that it is better to escape through the mind by reassuring the soul that it is safe to exist in the real world
- amnesia: provides the courage to deal with shocking past memories and face the world afresh
- anxiety: replaces unreasonable fear with a profound faith in the unlimited support of the universe
- apathy: instils enthusiasm and re-establishes a purpose for living
- Athlete's foot: clears the frustration of not speaking up for oneself or of allowing others to jump down one's throat by restoring one's belief in oneself
- bad breath (halitosis): purifies festering, revengeful, bitter, hurtful thoughts by improving inner communication through better understanding
- balance (loss of): centres the mind
- baldness: releases the intellect from the strain of doubt and uncertainty and eases the frustration of mentally 'pulling one's hair out'
- Bell's palsy: encourages the open expression of personal concepts
- bleeding gums: restores confidence and support in personal decisions
- blindness: replaces blinding fear through clearer vision and insight

- brain tumour: removes the malevolent growth of unexpressed disturbed, resentful thoughts making way for new, exciting concepts
- bruising: calms inner turmoil through greater self acceptance
- cancer: gets rid of contained upsetting thoughts and distressing emotions through compassion and comprehension so that they no longer get in the way of personal growth and development
- cataracts: enhances vision for a brighter outlook on life's prospects
- cerebral palsy: stimulates the thinking process for a more lively exchange of ideas
- cold sores: eliminates the festering need to 'give lip' or have to keep the 'lips sealed' by creating inner peace
- coma: provides loving acceptance of oneself and life in general
- conjunctivitis: soothes the anger and pain of all that seen or kept out of sight
- deafness: eliminates the fear of what is heard or not being heard
- depression: throws light on the meaning of life so that there is no longer a fear of being in the dark
- dizziness (vertigo): clarifies confused upsetting thoughts
- dry eyes: encourages the shedding of tears through greater understanding attained by seeing 'every point of view'
- earache: eases the pain and hurt of that which is being voiced or kept 'under the breath'
- epilepsy: dismisses the need to 'throw a fit' or 'bite one's tongue' by providing an opportunity to tune into a more acceptable wavelength whilst, at the same time, discovering ways in which to bring through one's extraordinary concepts
- eye disorders: improves insight for clearer vision so that disturbing events can be seen more clearly
- fainting: restores faith in the ability to cope and be in control
- gum disorders: strengthens and supports the basis of personal decisions
- headaches: eases the pain of everything coming to a head replacing it with a belief in one's ability to cope
- insomnia: soothes the mind so that body and soul can rest easily
- jaw disorders: reinstates faith in the foundation of personal concepts

- meningitis: dissipates contained anger and frustration arising from having to conceal or protect one's own unique notions
- migraine headaches: releases the mind from the intense pressure to perform
- mouth disorders: encourages open, honest communication within oneself
- nervousness: restores faith and belief in personal capabilities
- neuralgia: removes the pain and anguish of possible rejection or ridicule when communicating unusual ideas
- nose disorders: eliminates irritants that 'get up the nose' and prevents the nose from being 'knocked out of joint' through personal recognition of unique talents by ensuring that unusual ideas to be put into practice
- paralysis: frees the mind from gripping fear and enabling one's own ideas are mobilized for on-going progress
- Parkinson's disease: relinquishes the intense desire to organize or be organized by others through the re-establishment of inner control
- pituitary gland disorders: restores overall control and inner harmony
- seizures: dissipates profound frustration at not being understood
- sinus congestion: relieves accumulated irritability and the perceived need for everything to be perfect
- stroke: reduces self-inflicted pressure to meet unrealistically high expectations so that it is possible to get ahead with one's own personal concepts and ideas
- stuttering: boosts one's confidence in communicating and sharing personal concepts
- toothache: removes the agony and pain over decisions being made
- tinnitus: alerts the mind to the messages of the inner voice.

Reflexology massage of the toes

Massaging the toes, which contain the brain reflexes, has an immediate effect on the nervous system. This instantaneously encourages physical, mental, emotional and spiritual well-being. The resultant inner calm, peace and harmony ease the musculature, which makes it possible for all cells to receive essential life-forces so that they can function effectively and efficiently for the overall benefit of mind, body and soul. The way in which reflexology assists:

- relaxes, attunes and balances mind, body and soul
- makes space for rejuvenation and restoration by easing nervous tension
- encourages the natural functioning of all bodily parts, consciously, unconsciously and subconsciously.

Opening the energy flow

Opening the energy flow opens the mind, removes congestion from over-use of outdated belief systems and dispenses with fearful notions or frightful memories. This may cause the body to jerk and twitch as energy re-establishes its flow and life-force vibrancy gets through to previously deprived areas.

Step 1: opening the energy flow
- gently place each fingertip on top of all corresponding toes, excluding the big toes (Figure 26)
- slowly apply slight pressure for a few seconds
- gradually ease off until the fingertips are just resting on or hovering immediately above the skin's surface.

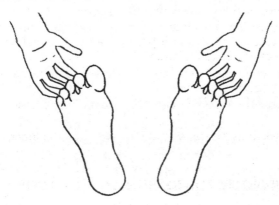

figure 26 opening the energy flow

Tingling or warmth felt between the fingers and toes is activated energy that revitalizes both recipient and the administrator.

Reconnecting with the Higher Self

By actively reconnecting with the super-consciousness of humanity, via our Higher Selves, we can attain greater understanding and compassion for fellow human beings, knowing that at soul level, although alone we are All One.

Step 2: reconnecting with the Higher Self
- remove all fingers and gently place the tips of the thumbs on top of the big toes (Figure 27)
- again, apply slight pressure, for a few seconds
- slowly ease off, until the fingertips just rest on or hover immediately above these toes.

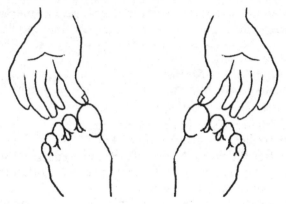

figure 27 reconnecting with the Higher Self

Brain, hair and sinus reflexes

The tips of the toes reflect the brain, hair and sinus reflexes (Figure 28). The brain represents the capacity to think, hair reflects the power of the mind whilst sinuses provide space to contemplate and play around with ideas. These reflexes are massaged (Figure 29) to put everything into perspective.

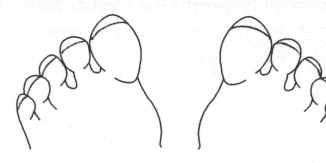

figure 28 brain, hair and sinus reflexes

Step 3: massaging the brain, hair and sinus reflexes

- place the little fingers on the outer edges of the little toes (Figure 29)
- slowly apply slight pressure for a few seconds
- then without moving the digits, gently rotate (see rotation movement on page 39)
- fractionally move the digits inwards
- repeat the rotation and continue until the tips of both little toes have been thoroughly massaged
- then place the fourth fingers on the outer edges of the fourth toes and repeat the sequence until the tips of both fourth toes have been thoroughly massaged
- repeat on the third toe with the third fingers, second toes with the index fingers and the big toes with the thumbs
- return to the outer edges of the little toes, this time with the little fingers fractionally lower down
- continue doing this technique in strips across the tips of all toes several times, each time finishing on the inner edge of both big toes.

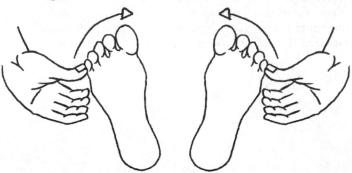

figure 29 massaging the brain reflexes

Massaging the brain reflexes:

- improves brain activity
- expands the capacity to think
- calms or excites the hypothalamus
- prolongs concentration
- alters thought patterns for a healthier state of mind, body and soul
- takes a weight off the mind
- provides space to contemplate new concepts for on-going growth and development.

Face reflexes

The face reflexes, situated on the toe pads of each toe, reveal how individuals face the world with their own unique concepts.

Step 4: massaging the face reflexes

- repeat the above sequence, from the outer edges of the little toe pads to the inner edges of the big toes
- if preferred the thumb can be used with the third fingers resting directly opposite on top of the toes instead of using the corresponding digits
- the dual use of digits can substantially increase the energy flow and so, if initially it proves too intense, keep the thumbs in position and remove the third fingers
- begin each strip fractionally further down the toe pads (Figure 30)
- continue until all toe pads have been thoroughly massaged.

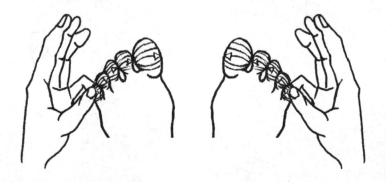

figure 30 massaging the face reflexes

Massaging the face reflexes:

- boosts self confidence
- eases confrontation
- assists in facing life situations
- enhances individual identity.

Remember to:

- spend time on 'congested' reflexes
- always massage the big toes particularly well since they contain the main head, brain and sensory reflexes
- the outer edges of each toe reflect the nerves, muscle, skin, bone, circulatory and lymphatic vessels of the sides of the face
- the inner surfaces mirror the inside core of the head, which contains the brain, pituitary gland, midbrain and cervical vertebrae as well nerves, muscle, skin, bone, circulatory and lymphatic vessels.

Forehead reflexes

The forehead reflexes (Figure 31) display the impression and expression of individual thoughts.

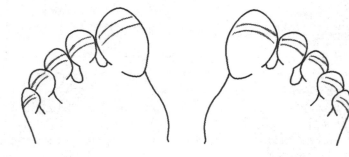

figure 31 forehead reflexes

Massaging the forehead reflexes:

- soothes the furrowed brow
- smoothes wrinkles of concern
- eases long-term anxiety.

Eye reflexes

The slight hollows above the mounds in the centres of all toe pads contain the eye reflexes (Figure 32).

The eyes are the 'windows to the soul', which reflect the mind's ability to focus and alter a multitude of light waves into meaningful shapes. They affect, and are affected by, all that is seen or not seen through the mind's eye. In this way perceptions and opinions are formed according to how much or how little one wishes to see, depending on current feelings and emotions.

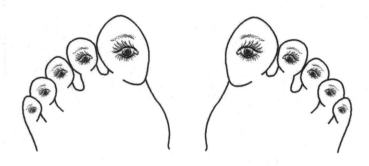

figure 32 eye reflexes

Step 5: massaging the eye reflexes

- gently place the thumbs on the centres of both little toe pads with the little fingers situated directly opposite on top of the little toes (Figure 33)
- lightly squeeze the two digits together
- when a slight resistance is felt hold for a few seconds
- then slowly rotate the thumbs
- gradually ease the compression until the digits barely touch the skin
- remove the thumbs then rest the little fingers on the centres of the little toe pads for a few seconds
- repeat on the fourth toe pads with the thumb and fourth fingers, then on the third with the thumb and third fingers and on the second toes with the thumbs and second fingers
- finally place the thumbs back on the big toe pads with the second fingers on top, squeeze release and balance

- visualization of the colour indigo whilst doing this intensifies the effect.

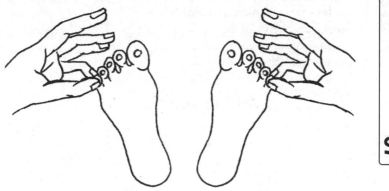

figure 33 massaging the eye reflexes

Massaging the eye reflexes:

- sharpens vision
- eases eye strain
- broadens personal outlook
- clarifies individual perceptions
- sharpens the focus
- maximizes optical functioning
- balances personal interpretation of environmental conditions.

Pineal gland reflexes

The pineal gland primary reflexes are the same as those of the pituitary gland (Figure 34) but they are more effectively accessed through their secondary reflexes, which they share with the eyes (Figure 32).

The pineal gland controls all natural cycles, such as mood cycles, sleep cycles, menstrual cycles and so on. It relies on the transmission of light waves that enter the body mainly through the eyes to function efficiently and produce the hormone melatonin. For this reason, the state and condition of the eyes are of utmost important because they reflect personal emotions and feelings, which have an immediate impact on the natural cycles of mind, body and soul according to what is being perceived.

Massaging the pineal gland:

- harmonizes natural cycles
- naturalizes the menstrual cycle
- stabilizes mood swings
- enhances intuition
- enlightens mind, body and soul.

Pituitary gland reflexes

Situated in the centre of the head beneath the hypothalamus of the brain is the pituitary gland, which is the master endocrine gland. Its reflexes are on the inner joints (big toe side) of all toes, especially the big toes (Figure 34).

The pituitary gland, like the conductor of the orchestra, instructs the rest of the endocrine glands when to function, the amount of hormone to provide, when to slow down and so on. Its role is to maintain inner harmony and accord throughout.

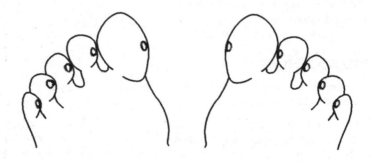

figure 34 pituitary gland reflexes

Step 6: massaging the pituitary gland reflexes

- lightly place the thumbs on the inner joints of both big toes (Figure 35)
- gradually apply gentle pressure whilst at the same time rotating
- ease the pressure
- remove the thumbs
- replace with the tips of the third fingers and lightly rest for a few seconds
- visualize the colour violet to enhance the effect.

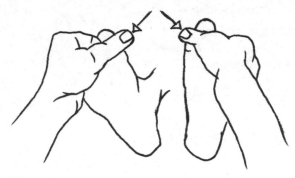

figure 35 massaging the pituitary gland reflexes

Massaging the pituitary gland reflexes:

- gives a clearer interpretation of messages from the hypothalamus
- calms the emotions
- creates inner harmony
- balances the secretion of hormones
- improves overall functioning of all endocrine glands.

Nose reflexes

The nose reflexes (Figure 36) arc the same as those for the pituitary gland (Figure 34).

The nose detects the most evocative of all senses, smell, which often brings to mind past memories associated with specific situations, people or events that either make 'one turn one's nose up' or revel in the aroma. The nose's capacity to function is affected by what is done or not done, hence common sayings such as 'putting one's nose into other people's business', which can 'get up one's nose' especially when being 'too nosy' or when ending up 'paying through the nose'. This is why the sense of smell heightens when on track and passionate about one's soul's purpose in life and the nose reflects recognition of oneself through personal success and achievements.

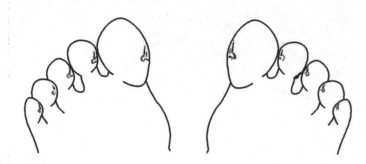

figure 36 nose reflexes

Massaging the nose reflexes:

- enhances the sense of smell
- encourages recognition of oneself
- gives one a nose for life
- keeps one on track with one's soul undertaking.

Ear reflexes

The ear reflexes are on the outer joints (little toe side) of all toes (Figure 37).

The ears represent the capacity to hear and really listen to what on earth is going on or not going on. Their reflexes reflect the precision with which sound waves are transformed into comprehensive signals to provide direction, guidance and balance, through the inner voice, of what to do and what not to do. It shows when information is 'going in one ear and out the other' or 'falling on deaf ears' from constantly receiving an 'earful' or when the ear has to be 'kept to the ground'.

Step 7: massaging the ear reflexes
- place the thumbs on the inner joints and the little fingers on the outer joints of both little toes (Figure 37)
- using the thumbs to support, massage with the little fingers, using the rotation movement
- then gently squeeze the digits together and apply slight pressure for a few seconds
- finally milk both sides of the toes from top to bottom with minimal compression between the digits

- repeat on the fourth toes with the thumb and fourth fingers, on the third toes with the thumb and third fingers, on the second toes with the thumb and second fingers, finishing on the big toes with the thumb and whichever digit feels most comfortable.

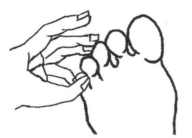 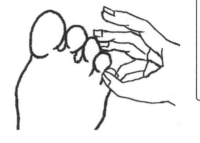

figure 37 massaging the ear reflexes

Massaging the ear reflexes:

- sharpens listening skills
- refines inner communication
- enhances the clarity of sounds
- clarifies the meaning of noises
- eases hearing disorders
- increases alertness
- improves balance
- facilitates understanding
- assists in accurate interpretation.

Mouth reflexes

The mouth reflexes (Figure 38) are immediately below the bony prominences of the nose and pituitary.

The mouth is directly involved in communications, the nature of which is affected by the type of personal relationship. This oral cavity is also actively involved in the intake and two-way exchange of life-force energies, in the form of nutrients and air. As the main connection between the internal and external worlds it influences and is influenced by on-going interactions or a lack thereof.

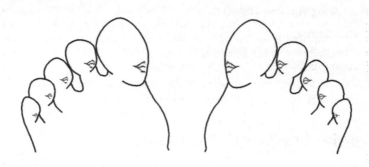

figure 38 mouth reflexes

Massage the mouth reflexes to:

- facilitate speech
- ease decision making
- enhance self-confidence
- increase security with personal concepts.

Jaw reflexes

The jaw reflexes (Figure 39) are situated along the lower edges of all toe pads.

The jaw provides a firm, mobile base to spring off ideas and perceptions. It reflects the degree of confidence when it comes to 'speaking one's mind'. Any uncertainty or fear of what others may think or say, however, causes many to hold back, which can build up causing an incredible amount of tautness in this area. For this reason, concentrate on massaging these reflexes well.

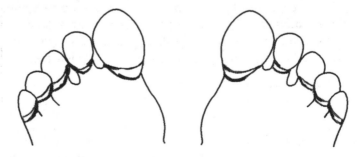

figure 39 jaw reflexes

Massaging the jaw reflexes:

- eases tension
- prevents tooth grinding
- boosts confidence in facing the world
- increases mobility for ideas to be expressed more freely
- enhances basic support for individual concepts.

Facial lymphatic reflexes

The concentration of lymphatic vessels and nodules in the head are reflected along both sides of each toe pad and toe neck (Figure 40).

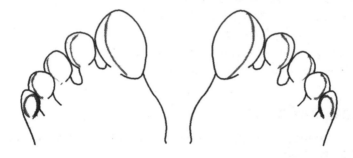

figure 40 facial lymphatic reflexes

Step 8: massaging the facial lymphatic reflexes

- place the thumb pads, one above the other, on the outer tip of the right little toe (Figure 41)
- soothingly, but firmly, stroke alternately with both thumbs (milking pages 40–1) in tiny movements from top to bottom
- repeat until the right little toe pad is thoroughly milked
- do the same on the fourth, third, second and big right toes
- then on the little, fourth, third, second and big left toes.

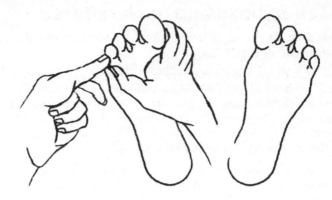

figure 41 massaging the facial lymphatic reflexes

Massaging the facial lymphatic reflexes:

- ensures a clear head
- opens the mind to every point of view
- removes emotional congestion
- soothes deeply ingrained impressions
- calms and reassures the mind
- clears the way for new concepts.

Face rejuvenation technique

Step 9: face rejuvenation technique

- 'feather stroke' (pages 41–2) the right little toe pad, then the fourth, third, second and big toes until all toe pads on the right foot have been soothed
- repeat on the left toe pads in the same sequence, starting on the left little toe and ending on the left big toe.

This light movement:

- lifts a weight off the mind
- creates space to think clearly
- raises the level of consciousness
- soothes the emotions
- establishes contact at soul level.

Back of head and neck reflexes

The back of the head and neck are reflected onto the upper surfaces of all toes.

The tops of the toes mirror the effect of thoughts tucked at the back of the mind, whilst the toe nails represent the skull, which protects the functioning of the brain and keeps it from harm or damage. In so doing it guards personal thoughts and ideas, especially from perceived criticism or mockery. This is reflected in the constantly changing characteristics of nails, which:

- thicken for additional protection, especially when outdated belief systems are desperately being hung on to
- become ridged in areas that need extra shielding (vertical ridges) or at times of vulnerability (horizontal ridges)
- lift or fall off to expose radical thoughts or 'from pulling one's hair out'.

Another way in which the body protects ideas and beliefs from coming under attack is to develop corns, which:

- on top of the toes, opposite the toe pad, appear to
  - stop others from 'walking over one's ideas'
  - avoid thoughts from being trampled upon
  - guard vulnerable, unthinkable notions
- appear on the toe necks to stop 'getting it in the neck' every time
  - one speaks up for oneself or
  - does not speak up and voice one's opinions
- appear on the outer edges (little toe side) when
  - 'turning a deaf ear'.

Step 10: massaging the back of the head and neck reflexes
- place four fingers on either side of both feet on the outer edges next to little toes
- move them in unison to 'walk' them over the tops of all the toes (Figure 42)
- finish on the inner edges of both big toes
- repeat two to three times.

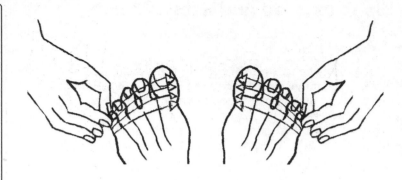

figure 42 massaging the back of the head and neck reflexes

Massaging the back of the head and neck reflexes:

- clears the clutter at the back of the mind
- eliminates fearful memories
- strengthens belief in personal concepts
- provides a firm backing for personal ideas
- opens the mind to every point of view.

Balancing mental energies

Balancing the mental energies ensures that the intellectual process is complemented by instinctive knowing for comprehensive insight, which ensures a more meaningful and manageable journey through life.

Step 11: balancing the mental energies

- lightly place the third fingers onto the tips of both little toes (Figure 43)
- rest them for a few seconds
- then move them onto the joints of the little toes
- stay a while before finally placing them at the bases of both little toes
- repeat on the fourth toes, third toes, second toes and lastly the big toes.

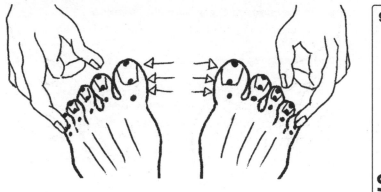

figure 43 balancing the mental energies

Balancing the mental energies:

- increases the energy flow to and from the brain
- clears mental congestion
- eases cranial pressure
- relaxes the neck muscles
- improves circulation between the brain and the rest of the body.

Midbrain reflexes

The midbrain is reflected onto the outer edges of both big toes, immediately above the bony joint (Figure 44).

The midbrain is responsible for synchronized muscular movements as well as the breathing and circulation processes since it also contains the cardiac and respiratory centres.

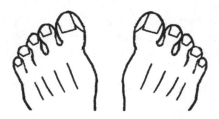

figure 44 midbrain reflexes

Step 12: massaging the midbrain reflexes

- place the thumbs or fingers on the tips of both big toes (Figure 45)
- gently massage the small strip on the edge of the toes as far as the joints on the outside edges
- repeat several times moving the digit a fraction either way of the strip to make the area slightly wider
- milk with tiny soothing strokes (pages 40–1)
- then feather stroke(pages 41–2) .

Massaging the midbrain reflexes:

- fine tunes muscular co-ordination
- improves respiration
- enhances cardiac and circulatory functioning
- encourages a balanced approach to life.

Spinal reflexes

The bony vertebrae of the spine are reflected along the hard ridges of bone that extend from the joints along the outer edges of both big toes to beneath the inner ankles (Figure 45).

The spinal reflexes reflect one's innate ability to provide solid support and backing for mind, body and soul (Figure 45).

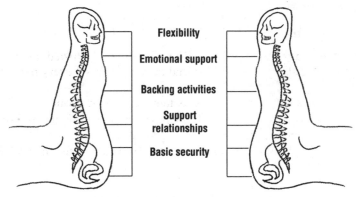

figure 45 spinal reflexes

Step 13: massaging the spinal reflexes

- place the thumbs or fingers on the inner joints of both big toes (Figure 47)

- gently massage the length of both bony ridges that border the central portion of the feet finishing by going beneath both inner ankle-bones
- repeat with the thumbs angled onto the top of the bony ridge to stimulate or calm the sensory nerves
- then do this again, but this time with the thumbs gently pushing upwards underneath the bony ridge to balance the motor nerves
- milk with small, repetitive soothing strokes from toe to ankle, first on the right spinal reflex and then on the left reflex
- feather stroke in the same way with an exceptionally light touch.

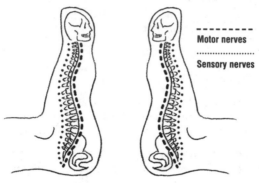

figure 46 massaging the spinal reflexes

Massaging the spinal reflexes:

- soothes agitated nerves and/or stimulates petrified nerves, affecting all systems since spinal nerves infiltrate every part of the body
- facilitates the relay of nervous messages throughout
- increases and alerts each cell's awareness of its bodily environment
- improves overall functioning for optimum efficiency and effectiveness.

Metamorphic technique

Finally in this section, the Metamorphic technique liberates past fears and anxieties, especially those experienced whilst in the womb.

- the tips of the big toes represent the point of conception
- the spinal reflexes reflect the time in the womb
- the ankle represents the time of birth (Figure 47).

Step 14: the metamorphic technique

- lightly place the tips of the third fingers on top of both big toes
- keep them still for a few seconds
- then barely touching the skin's surface, slide the fingers slowly over the spinal reflexes under the inner ankles finishing at the back of these bony protrusions
- remain here for a few seconds before repeating the stroking movement two to three more times
- a tiny circular movement can also be used along the spinal reflexes in conjunction with the above.

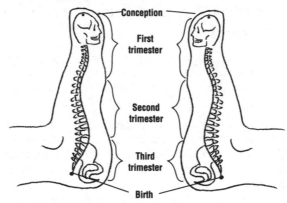

figure 47 reflections of time in the womb

The metamorphic technique:

- unlocks and releases fearful memories of one's time in the womb
- assists in cutting the invisible umbilical cord between parent and offspring
- re-establishes an innate knowing of oneself.

The arches

The condition of the arches, the bony insteps, reflects inner strength and the perceived amount of backing and support according to whether one is happy about being 'in step' or feeling 'out of step' with general belief systems.

Arches are greatly affected by all that is believed 'to be going on behind one's back' and by all that 'the back has been turned on'.

- babies lack insteps due to their total dependence on the support of others, until increased confidence and personal development encourages them to 'stand on their own two feet'
- once developed the instep should remain stable and supportive
- flat feet occur when there is
  - extreme emotional strain causes the arch to collapse
  - no perceived need to 'stand up for oneself'
- over-extended arches indicate
  - the need for extra support and backing
  - 'bending over backwards' to please others.

Effect of reflexology on the head, face and spinal reflexes

Massaging the toes, with the head and face reflexes, and the bony insteps, which reflect the spine, has far-reaching effects due to their relationship with the nervous system. Nerves infiltrate the whole body making it a sensitive, responsible being.

Reflexology either stimulates or pacifies the nerves, which immediately affects reactions and functioning of the corresponding parts throughout the whole body. Furthermore, it encourages a change of mind encouraging a more meaningful approach to life in the following ways:

- calms the nerves
- clarifies and strengthens the relationship between the brain and the rest of the body
- improves concentration
- raises the level of consciousness
- clarifies perception
- fine tunes the senses, particularly intuition
- heightens natural sensitivity
- creates a harmonious inner environment
- boosts self-worth
- balances the level of tolerance
- incites healthy actions and reactions
- enhances internal and external relationships
- improves muscular co-ordination
- encourages overall well-being and general health.

Summary of the toes

Massage of the individual sets of toes:

- big toes: stimulates intellect and intuition, clarifying thoughts by enhancing personal beliefs and convictions in one's own individual unique and innovative ideas
- second toes boosts perception of self-esteem and self-worth
- third toes: encourages and inspires innovative ideas to be put into practice for the production of on-going constructive and worthwhile notions
- fourth toes: allows new concepts to enliven personal ways of communicating
- little toes: expands and frees the mind from inhibiting belief systems and social restraints allowing more extraordinary ideas to lead the way.

In between each sequence

Massage each foot individually, from top to bottom, to enhance the overall effect of each sequence.

Cup the right foot between both hands and stroke from the toes to the ankles and around the heels, two to three times (Figure 48) and then repeat on the left foot.

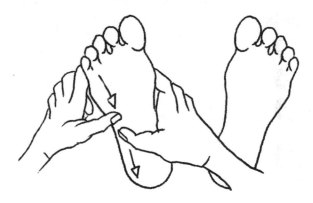

figure 48 massaging in between sequences

We are what we think.

08

big toes and toe necks

In this chapter you will ascertain:
- that the big toes reflect the mind, which is the key to overall healing.

Big toes

The big toes mirror the main reflexes for:

- head
- brain
- face
- cranium.

They reflect:

- thoughts
- ideas
- intellect
- intuition
- spirituality
- Higher Self.

The reflexes are related to the:

- toe necks
- thumbs.

The associated systems are:

- nervous
- endocrine
- sensory
- lymphatic.

Specific characteristics:

- represent ether
- resonate to indigo, violet, purple and white.

The big toes contain the main head and brain reflexes, the expression of which is dependent on the neck and throat, which are reflected in the toe necks. These reveal the two-way exchange of life-force energies from the non-physical to the physical and vice versa. The condition of the toe necks depends on honest, open expression between the inner and outer worlds.

Natural characteristics of the big toes and toe necks

In their natural state the big toes and toe necks should stand supply upright and be firm, but flexible, with smooth, pliable, flesh-coloured skin.

Impact of tension on the thought process and expression of personal concepts and ideas

Terror of standing up for oneself and putting one's own ideas into practice for fear of the frightful consequences causes anxiety, concern and worry. The more an individual succumbs to other belief systems, to the detriment of one's own brilliant concepts, allowing oneself to be conditioned into prescribed ways of thinking, the worse the situation becomes.

Not being in control leads to a righteous approach and, ironically, the increasing incidence of 'control freak-ism'. The more out of control we are, the more we try to control! This is contributing to the increase in nervous dis-orders, which is 'stopping many in their tracks' through strokes, Parkinson's disease, brain tumours or head injuries.

Furthermore, fear of 'speaking up for oneself' and voicing one's own unique concepts clamps down on the throat and neck muscles, effectively choking and throttling personal individuality. Dread of speaking up arises from:

- apprehension of ridicule
- terror of the consequences
- concern about outside opinion
- trepidation of upsetting others.

When personal creativity is strangled and stifled by social restraints, restrictions and expectations, it can lead to anger, guilt or stubbornness, causing:

- lumps of unleashed emotion
- post-natal drip, from swallowing tears from fear of openly crying
- sore throats from the pain and strain of trying to disclose true feelings

- inflammation from swallowing or shouting angry, infuriating words.

Feeling insecure about expressing one's own ideas and feelings, tenses neck muscles and reduces agility. This may result in:

- a pain in the neck due to personal beliefs being threatened
- spasm from fear
- stabbing pains from 'getting it in the neck'.

Altered states of the big toes and toe necks

The stature and state of the big toes immediately reveal whether an individual is on track with their own ideas and soul purpose, in the following ways:

- bend to the side, crushing the other toes succumbing to alien beliefs whilst suppressing one's own ideas and/or putting them to one side
- bow in subservience to please others or 'bow out' of facing the world with one's extraordinary ideas
- sink into their socket, when under another's thumb
- rigidify due to a dogmatic and unbending approach because of set beliefs and ideas.

Difficulty in expressing the true self is reflected in the toe necks in the following ways:

- creases and wrinkles from strain, concern and worry
- distinct lines across the throat reflexes from feeling throttled
- lumps when feeling choked with emotion
- swellings on outside edges (little toe sides) from post-nasal drip, the swallowed tears of suppressed emotions
- weeping from extreme sadness and drowning in sorrow.

Skin colouring (pages 71–2) provides further clues as to the sentiment behind the expression of life or feelings at being prevented from openly divulging oneself.

- red from frustration, anger or embarrassment
- white from exhaustion or enlightenment
- blue or black when hurt
- yellow from being fed up or energised
- green from envy or passion.

Neck and throat dis-orders relieved through reflexology

Regardless of the dis-orders, a complete reflexology massage is always required, with specific attention to:

- the nervous system and solar plexus reflexes to calm the mind and relieve pain, anxiety and fear
- the endocrine gland reflexes to soothe the emotions and create inner harmony
- the affected gland or organ reflexes to relax the distressed area and ease the symptoms of distress.

The way in which reflexology relieves these dis-orders is as follows:

- goitre: reduces the need to outwardly project oneself by openly recognizing one's unique way of articulating oneself
- hyperthyroidism: makes space for self-expression
- hypothyroidism: boosts self-confidence and re-energizes the whole
- laryngitis: pacifies inflamed, angry and frustrated expressions that have been swallowed and are festering in the throat
- lump in the throat: provides the inner resourcefulness to deal with perceivably adverse or traumatic situations
- neck problems: eases rigidity and tension through greater flexibility so that every point of view can be considered
- post-nasal drip: releases swallowed tears of joy, pride or grief allowing them to flow freely
- sore throat: eliminates the hurt of not being heard and encourages the individual to speak up for themselves
- stiff neck: removes 'the blinkers' so that life can be viewed from many different angles and points of view
- tonsillitis: re-establishes belief in personal creativity and opens the way for the free flow of complete individuality.

Throat reflexes

The surfaces of all toe necks, above the soles of the feet, reflect the throat (Figure 49).

The right toe necks mirror the right side of the throat revealing the effect of past expressions, whilst the left side of the throat rebounds on the left toe necks to show the exchange of life's expressions in the present.

Step 1: massaging the throat reflexes

- place both thumbs on the outer edges of the little toe necks with the third fingers directly opposite on top of the little toe necks (Figure 49)
- gently squeeze the corresponding digits together and then slowly release until there is only slight contact
- lightly rotate the thumbs (pages 38–9), whilst resting the third fingers on top
- move the thumbs fractionally along the little toe necks, still with the third fingers directly opposite, on top
- repeat the gentle squeezing, release and rotation technique until the little toe necks and then all toe necks are completely massaged
- concentrate on the sides of each toe where the greatest tension and emotional congestion are often reflected
- follow this sequence for as long as required.

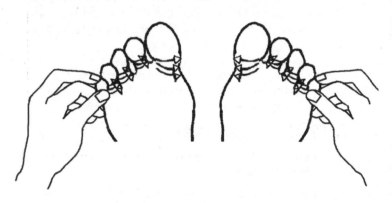

figure 49 massaging the throat reflexes

Massaging the throat reflexes:

- eases throat congestion
- reduces cerebral tension
- increases blood flow to and from the head
- assists lymphatic activity
- opens avenues of expression.

Step 2: milking the throat reflexes

- use the thumbs to gently, but firmly, stroke and milk the underneath surface of the toe necks, from top to bottom (pages 40–1), starting on the little toes necks and finishing on the big toe necks (Figure 50)
- then feather stroke (pages 41–2) in the same way.

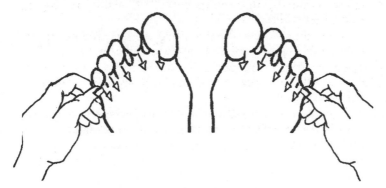

figure 50 massaging the throat reflexes downwards

Milking the neck reflexes:

- facilitates internal and external expression.

Thyroid gland reflexes

The thyroid gland is reflected onto the lower, inner creases of the necks of both big toes (Figure 51).

The thyroid gland reflexes mirror the innate need, to spread one's wings and be free of any constraints or restrictions, as their butterfly shape suggests.

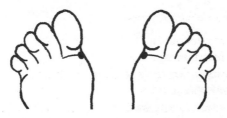

figure 51 thyroid gland reflexes

These expressive reflexes:

- distend: to reach out for more time and space for oneself
- diminish: when exhausted from doing so much for others
- harden: when there's a resistance to one's own opinions
- develop a layer of hard skin to protect individuality.

Step 3: massaging the thyroid gland reflexes

- lightly place the thumbs on both creases at the bases on the inside edges of the big toes (Figure 52) with the second fingers placed directly above on top of the feet
- gently squeeze the digits together and hold
- ease the pressure
- then lightly rotate the thumbs for a few seconds
- remove the thumbs and rest the tips of the second fingers on both reflexes, barely touching the skin's surface
- stay in this position, without movement, for a while, to balance the gland
- soothingly stroke the reflexes
- visualize turquoise/blue to enhance the effect.

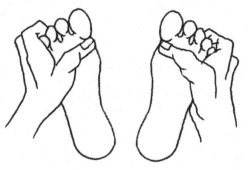

figure 52 massaging the thyroid gland reflexes

Massaging the thyroid gland reflexes:

- reduces the need to be continually on top of situations
- restores faith when tempted to give in
- balances metabolism
- provides space to just be oneself.

Shoulder reflexes

The shoulders are reflected onto the upper portion of both balls of the feet, immediately beneath the toe necks.

These reflexes reveal an individual's innate ability, willingness or strength in carrying on regardless of variable circumstances within the emotional environment.

These reflexes swell to show:

- the burdens of responsibility
- defence through hunching in an attempt to avoid taking on too much.

They sink when:

- tired of carrying hefty burdens or so many issues
- giving in under the strain of having to take on so much
- weighed down by having so much on one's shoulders.

Step 4: massaging the shoulder reflexes

- place the thumbs on the outer edges of both balls of the feet, immediately below the little toes, with the third fingers situated directly above, on top of the feet (Figure 53)
- gently squeeze the corresponding digits together
- apply slight pressure and then release.
- without moving position, lightly rotate the thumbs (pages 38–9) whilst the third fingers continue to rest gently on top
- move all digits along the horizontal strips, beneath the necks of the little toes, and repeat the squeeze, release, rotation movement
- continue as far as the big toes
- massage these strips several times, especially if they are hard or swollen.

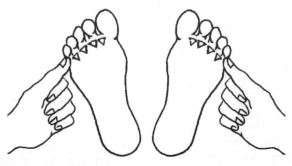

figure 53 massaging the shoulder reflexes

Massaging the shoulder reflexes:

- takes a 'weight off the shoulders'
- eases the perceived need to 'shoulder responsibilities'
- enhances blood flow to and from the head, specifically to the ears and eyes.

Step 5: milking the shoulder reflexes

- stroke or milk (pages 40–1) by sliding the thumbs firmly, but gently, along the bases of the little toe necks (Figure 54)
- then slide them through the gaps between the little and fourth toes
- continue along the bases of the fourth toe necks and into the gaps between the fourth and third toes
- repeat beneath the third and second toe necks finishing in the gaps between the second and big toes
- redo several times as required.

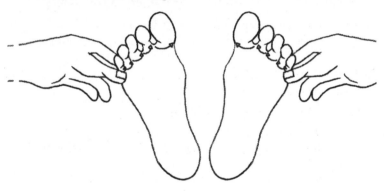

figure 54 milking the shoulder reflexes

Milking the shoulder reflexes:

- relaxes the clavicle bones
- expands the chest
- improves stature.

Upper arm reflexes

The upper arm reflexes extend from the protruding bones, underneath the little toes, on top of both feet, along the ridge of bone on the outer edges of the balls of the feet, to the bony protrusion, midway down the outer edges (Figure 55).

These reflexes mirror the following parts:

- the protruding bones reflect the shoulder sockets
- the ridges of bone represent the upper arms
- the midway bony protrusions mirror the elbow reflexes.

The upper arm reflexes reflect the amount of personal freedom to be oneself and the ability to expand and fully embrace the wholeness of life.

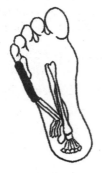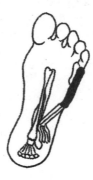

figure 55 upper arm reflexes

The characteristics of these reflexes are influenced in the following ways:

- they swell when trying to break free from:
  - unreasonable restraints
  - inhibiting or overwhelming emotions, especially within the family
  - an emotionally fraught environment
- they develop hard skin over the swelling to cover up and conceal one's true emotions.

Step 6: massaging the upper arm reflexes

- place the thumbs or the second fingers immediately below the little toes
- massage thoroughly either with the caterpillar or rotation movements (pages 38–40) to the prominent bones midway down the outer edges
- then milk (pages 40–1) and finally feather stroke (pages 41–2).

Massaging the upper arm reflexes:

- releases the individual from self-imposed restraints that pin them down
- provides the strength to reach out for meaningful experiences.

Neck reflexes

The cervical vertebrae are reflected along the bony inner edges of both big toes whilst the rest of the neck is reflected along the tops of each toe neck.

These bony structures mirror the following:

- degree of flexibility available to pivot the head and see every point of view
- amount of backing and support available for honest, open expression.

Rigidity in these reflexes indicates extreme anxiety and uncertainty in speaking up for oneself or a set determination to stick one's neck out.

Step 7: massaging the neck reflexes

- place four fingers either side of the feet on the little toe necks (Figure 56)
- move them in unison to 'walk' over the tops of all the toes
- finish on the inner edges of the necks of the big toes
- repeat two to three times
- milk (pages 40–1) and feather stroke (pages 41–2).

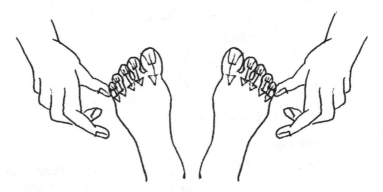

figure 56 massaging the neck reflexes

Massaging the neck reflexes:

- eases neck tension
- relaxes neck muscles
- increases flexibility.

Influence of reflexology on the big toes and toe necks

The reflexology massage reflectively:

- reconnects the individual with their soul purpose
- raises consciousness
- soothes and relaxes neck and throat muscles
- creates space for the free flow and exchange of energies to and from the brain
- opens the avenues of expression
- eases internal and external communication.

In between each sequence

Gently caress the tops of the feet by lightly running the tips of all fingers from the tips of the toes to the ankles (Figure 57) to soothe evoked memories that have been tucked behind one's back.

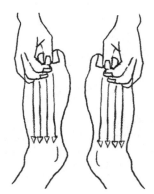

figure 57 soothing the nerves

Stroke both feet a few times, from the top to bottom (Figure 48) and then move onto massaging the balls of the feet (pages 112–35).

Something we withhold makes us afraid and weak, until we find that it is ourselves!

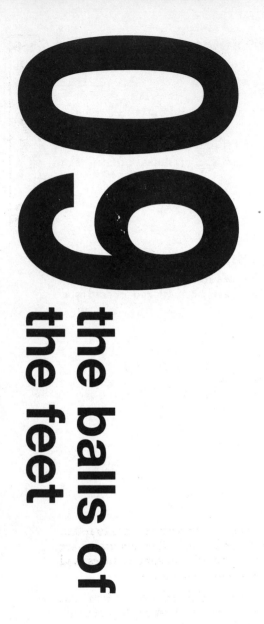

09

the balls of the feet

In this chapter you will see:
- how the balls of the feet mirror feelings and emotions that are the impetus to drive us into action.

The balls of the feet mirror the:

- shoulders
- chest
- breast
- ribcage
- lungs
- thymus gland
- upper arms
- airways
- oesophagus
- upper back.

They reflect:

- feelings of self-esteem
- internal emotions.

The reflexes are related to the:

- second toes
- second fingers
- eyes
- elbows
- knees.

The associated systems are:

- respiratory system
- cardiac and circulatory system.

Specific characteristics:

- represent air
- resonate to green and pink.

The balls of the feet reflect the chest and breast reflexes to reveal feelings of self-esteem and self-worth. These then determine the way individuals relate and respond to constant changes and fluctuations with their emotional environment.

Our first breath at birth is our initial act of freedom and independence, with our very presence demanding space be made for each of us to be an individual in our own right.

From then onwards, fresh supplies of vital life-force energies reinforce these feelings according to our emotional environment since our emotions either inflate or deflate our perception of ourselves and others. This, in turn determines the amount of air taken in from the surrounding atmosphere for the beneficial functioning and participation of mind, body and soul.

Once the advantageous aspects of inhaled air have been realized and utilized, the by-product, carbon dioxide, is immediately eliminated. This is to prevent it from accumulating and threatening personal well-being since it is symbolic of worked through emotions that, if retained, could be a potential threat and cause serious harm to personal well-being.

Within a harmonious, happy environment, lungs have an incredible capacity to expand and contract rhythmically. This encourages a healthy balance between the on-going acceptance of the many beneficial aspects of life, whilst, at the same time, refusing to admit potentially invasive substances.

This process is either enhanced or hampered by self-esteem. Crushing feelings of defeat and futility deflate the whole, whilst boosted morale substantially expands the chest.

The exchange of life-forces is also directly related to the nurturing process via the breasts, the characteristics and size of which change continually according to the amount of loving care being given and received.

Natural characteristics of the balls of the feet

The balls of the feet are naturally flesh-coloured mounds that occupy the upper third of the soles, immediately below the toe necks.

Their flexibility and colour reflect an individual's ability to adapt comfortably and blend into any environment, as well as to variations within emotional circumstances.

Altered states of the balls of the feet

The constant variation of colours on the balls of the feet reveal fluctuating emotions that are jogged as thoughts move through the body hence the word 'emotion' i.e. 'e' = 'energy' which is thought, that is in 'motion'.

- red indicates embarrassment, frustration or inflamed emotions
- white suggests being: drained of energy, tired and exhausted, or being enlightened
- various shades of blue to black display varying degrees of deep hurt and bruised feelings
- yellow occurs when either feeling fed up or needing to do something more worthwhile to feel better
- green is evidence of envy or reveals the need for space or possibly the need to outwardly display one's overwhelming love.

Noticing changes of colours over specific reflexes on the balls of the feet provides invaluable insight into innermost sensations that affect the whole.

Respiratory, circulatory, breast and immunity dis-orders

Respiratory disorders occur when:

- there is diminished interest in life
- feeling inadequate
- emotionally disillusioned
- feeling deflated
- heartfelt opinions are kept close to the chest
- true sentiments are concealed behind a smoke screen
- unable to breathe for oneself.

Circulatory dis-eases occur when:

- feeling a failure
- not able to circulate due to a lack of self-esteem and self-worth
- greed and insensitivity take over
- heartbreaking situations are allowed to linger
- everything is 'taken too much to heart'.

Breast complications are evidence of:

- being drained and exhausted from nurturing others
- creativity and individuality being stifled
- feeling emotionally abandoned or cut-off
- feeling suffocated by overwhelming situations.

Immunity issues arise when:

- attacking oneself and/or others for not being 'good enough'
- feeling vulnerable and under attack
- feeling defenceless
- have no perceivable 'leg to stand on'.

Respiratory, cardiac, breast and immunity dis-orders relieved through reflexology

Regardless of the dis-order, a complete reflexology massage is always required, with specific attention to the:

- nervous system and solar plexus reflexes to calm the mind and relieve any pain, anxiety and fear
- endocrine gland reflexes to soothe the emotions and create inner harmony
- affected gland or organ reflexes to relax the distressed area and ease the symptoms of distress.

Reflexology assists specific ailments in the following ways:

- aids: replaces feelings of inadequacy with enhanced belief in oneself and one's unique individuality and value in society
- allergies: eases extreme irritability and vulnerability by increasing or decreasing the level of tolerance by soothing excessive sensitivity
- anaemia: replenishes inner strength by boosting self-worth
- arteries: relaxes the blood vessels so that they can become filled with renewed enthusiasm and lovingly nurture all cells for on-going personal growth and development
- arteriosclerosis: releases the arteries from perceived pressures and removes the need to develop hardened resistance by reinstating an innate trust in the life process
- asphyxiating attacks: reduces the panic of being overwhelmed and suffocated by encouraging a more expansive acceptance of all that comes one's way
- asthma, removes the panic of feeling smothered, overprotected or overwhelmed by dissipating suffocating emotions and by making space for the individual to breath on their own

- bleeding: replaces deep sadness with greater understanding, love and joy
- blood pressure: maintains a harmonious flow of love and joy throughout
- high blood pressure: dissolves unresolved emotional issues so that blood vessels can expand and embrace new beginnings
- low blood pressure: re-establishes the flow of passion and delight by enhancing self-acceptance
- blood disorders: ensures inner harmony for the unimpeded flow of happiness
- blood clotting: opens channels of communication so that they remain viable
- breast cysts: contained emotions of extreme frustration from either not receiving enough or giving too much nurturing are made increasingly manageable
- breathing disorders: feelings of inadequacy are eliminated, creating space for improved self-esteem to inflate the whole
- bronchitis: frustration and anger at personal wellbeing being threatened within the environment are put into proportion
- bunions: entrapped, contained emotions become liberated
- carpal tunnel syndrome: distress about the way in which life is being handled is eased
- circulation: inner peace and unconditional acceptance of oneself enhance the flow and distribution of life-forces for overall nurturing
- cholesterol: faith in the loving process is reinstated as the gripping fear or distrust of emotional commitment dissipates
- colds: repressed irritability of all that has got 'up one's nose' is unleashed, making way for the beginning of an exciting new cycle
- congestion: perceived obstacles dissipate so that the natural flow of life-forces is enhanced throughout
- emphysema: belief in oneself is boosted for the courage to live life to the full
- heartburn: the gripping fear of heartfelt issues becomes less threatening
- hyperventilation: inner panic is calmed
- increased blood acidity: bitterness at the lack of love and joy diminishes as the good things in life become more apparent

- increased white blood cells: the body naturally fortifies itself, especially during periods of perceived personal abuse and attack
- knee disorders: previously unwelcome changes in direction are facilitated for greater progress to be made
- leukaemia: the soul is liberated from unexpressed resentment at the lack of love arising from unrealistic pressures and expectation
- lung disorders: the whole is filled with an appreciation of the self for inner contentment and an enhanced relationship within the environment
- mastitis: anger and frustration at the emotional demands of others dissipate and are replaced with feelings of personal appreciation
- pneumonia: emotional hurts heal to allow the whole to be filled with exuberance
- round shoulders: perceived burdens of responsibility are lifted from the shoulders so that appropriate emotional responses can be made
- sickle cell anaemia: room becomes available for pure love and understanding through the removal of social restraints and restrictions that previously inhibited the flow
- thymus disorders: vulnerability is reduced and inner strength reinforced through the belief that nothing and no-one is a threat unless allowed to be
- upper back discomfort: emotional backing and support are strengthened through non-critical acceptance of the self
- varicose veins: the weight and burdens of disagreeable circumstances, which are generally accompanied by hopeless discouragement, are replaced with greater understanding and a renewed enthusiasm to go with the flow of life.

Lung reflexes

The lungs are reflected onto the balls of both feet and occupy the bulk of this area, top and bottom (Figure 58).

Lungs represent the ability to take in expansive breaths of life to boost one's belief in oneself. Interference of this process is reflected onto the balls of the feet:

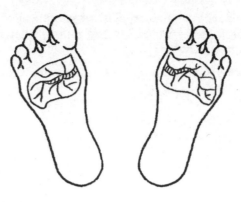

figure 58 lung reflexes

Lung reflexes:

- enlarge when
  - weighed down with hefty emotions
  - breath-taking feelings are kept close to the chest
  - giving away too much of oneself
  - feeling that others are taking advantage
  - reaching out for love and affection

- flatten when
  - feeling winded
  - feeling deflated
  - drained of self nourishment
  - lacking self-esteem
  - being denied loving feelings

- wrinkle when
  - concerned about what others are feeling
  - worried about the emotional environment
  - feeling crushed

- develop marks, which highlight
  - the impact of heartfelt emotions that have left their mark
  - deep impressions made on one's personality

- develop lines, which indicate
  - divided loyalties
  - completely different emotional environments

- develop hard skin and calluses, which appear to
  - protect, shield and/or conceal feelings that may drain or threaten self-worth.

Step 1: horizontal massage of the lung reflexes

- place the thumbs on the outer edges of both balls of the feet, immediately below the shoulder reflexes (Figure 59) with the second fingers situated directly above
- gently squeeze the corresponding digits together
- apply slight pressure and then release
- staying in the same position, lightly rotate the thumbs (pages 38–9) with the second finger still resting on top
- move the thumbs fractionally along the horizontal strip with the second fingers following
- repeat the squeeze, release and rotation movement
- continue along the width of the balls of both feet to the inside edges, beneath the big toes
- return to the outer edges of both balls of the feet, this time placing the digits fractionally lower down
- continue the horizontal massage across the balls of the feet until both are thoroughly massaged.

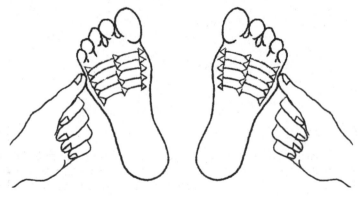

figure 59 massaging the lung reflexes (1)

Step 2: vertical massage of the lung reflexes

- again place the thumbs on the balls of both feet beneath the little toes (Figure 60)
- either caterpillar (pages 39–40) or rotate (pages 38–9) the thumbs in vertical strips from top to the bottom

- continue until the balls of both feet have been thoroughly massaged
- milk (page 40) with the thumbs from top to bottom
- then feather stroke (page 41) very lightly with the second fingers in the same direction.

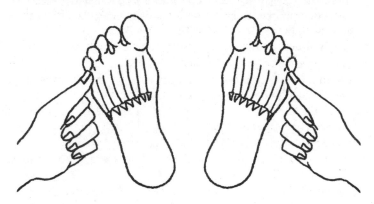

figure 60 massaging the lung reflexes (2)

Massaging the lung reflexes:

- creates spaces to breathe
- inflates feelings of well being
- encourages self-enhancement
- assists effortless adaptation to constantly changing emotional environments
- facilitates the exchange of life-force energies.

Breast reflexes

The breast reflexes overlap the lung reflexes in the balls of the feet and can be accessed either from the soles (primary reflexes) (Figure 61) or from the corresponding areas on top of the feet (secondary reflexes).

The breasts display an individual's ability to provide amply for themselves, as well as nurture the essence within. The size of breasts, especially on females, indicates the amount of nurturing to oneself and others:

- large bosoms have a tremendous capacity to nurture but tend to give away too much of themselves, resulting in the need to reach out for more affection for themselves
- flattened mammary glands indicate being completely drained and exhausted from caring so much for others to the detriment of oneself, or they suggest that the individual is withholding the nurturing process from themselves because they do not feel good enough.

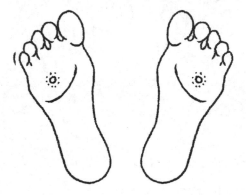

figure 61 breast reflexes

Massaging the breast reflexes:

- ensures that there is adequate substance for all concerned
- eases emotional congestion
- facilitates the nurturing process
- eliminates resentment and anger at the lack of nurturing or over protection
- assists in finding a balance in the give and take of nurturing issues.

Thymus gland reflexes

The thymus gland reflexes are on the inner edges halfway down the balls of both feet (Figure 62).

The thymus gland represents the seat of the soul. Its reflexes feel:

- slightly swollen in the very young, elderly and during vulnerable phases
- hollow in older children, teenagers and adults.

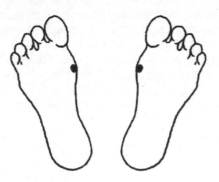

figure 62 thymus reflexes

When an individual feels under attack the thymus gland produces killer T-cells, which sadly destroy its own body, highlighting feelings of being soul destroyed. Unnatural thymus reflex characteristics include:

- bunions that develop in an attempt to break free from stifling emotions that entrap the soul and rob it of its individuality
- swellings over the reflexes when reaching out for personal recognition
- hard skin that forms as a shield to protect, conceal or cover up personal feelings especially when feeling vulnerable
- subsidence from the exhaustion of defending oneself from emotional abuse and perceived criticism.

Step 3: massaging the thymus reflexes
- place the thumbs halfway down the inner edges of both balls of the feet with the second fingers resting directly opposite on the tops of the feet (Figure 63)
- feel either for slight hollows or possible swellings (see page 122)
- gently squeeze the digits together and hold for a few seconds
- slightly release the pressure
- lightly rotate (pages 38–9) the thumbs without moving position with the second fingers still resting on top
- stop rotating and hold, without moving, for a few seconds
- remove the thumbs and lightly rest the tips of the second fingers on the reflexes for a while
- gently stroke with the second fingers
- visualize green to enhance the effect.

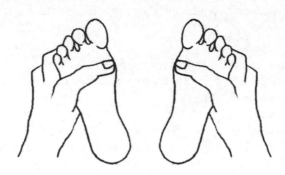

figure 63 massaging the thymus reflexes

Massaging the thymus reflexes:

- boosts self-esteem and self-worth
- eases soul-destroying events such as a broken relationship, death, and retrenchment
- strengthens immunity.

Heart reflexes

The heart is reflected onto the inside edges, where the balls of the feet and insteps meet. The reflex is larger on the left foot because of the heart's position in the body (Figure 64).

The heart is the centre of love and joy that delights in nourishing and caring for all the body's cells. It relies on complete acceptance of oneself and others in order to function at its best.

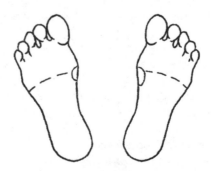

figure 64 heart reflexes

Heart rendering situations affect the heart and heart reflexes can:

- enlarge when
  - overwhelmed by heartfelt issues
  - reaching out for pure love and affection
- fade when feeling
  - drained
  - disillusioned with the process of love.
- miniscule blood blisters may develop when broken hearted
- hard skin forms when
  - perceivably under attack
  - trying to conceal one's heartfelt emotions
- cut due to feeling
  - cut off, usually after a divorce or separation
  - split and torn apart.

Step 4: massaging the heart reflexes

- lightly place the tips of the second and third fingers on the heart reflexes (Figure 65)
- apply slight pressure for a while and then slowly ease off
- gently rotate the digits for a few seconds
- stop the movements
- rest the second then the third fingers on both reflexes
- lovingly stroke these sensitive reflexes
- visualize green and/or pink to enhance the effect.

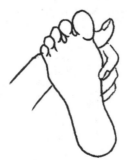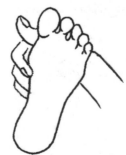

figure 65 massaging the heart reflexes

Massaging the heart reflexes:

- strengthens and purifies affections
- opens the heart to pure love for oneself and others.

Circulation is life, stagnation is death.

Oesophagus reflexes

The oesophagus reflexes extend from the mouth reflexes, on the pads of the big toes, along the inner edges of the toe necks onto the balls of both feet to where they meet with the fleshy instep (Figure 66).

The oesophagus represents the ability to ingest life's events according to what is on the mind and how well one is feeling about everything that is being taken in on a daily basis.

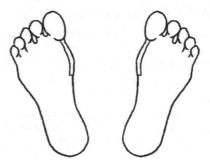

figure 66 oesophagus reflexes

Unusual reflexes include:

- a ridge of hard skin develops
  - when life is hard to swallow
  - to conceal true feelings regarding life's circumstances
- noticeable colour changes
  - white when tired of having things 'thrust down one's throat'
  - red due to being angry, frustrated or embarrassed at having to swallow certain situations
  - blue from hurt at being taken in

- flaky skin indicating
  - irritability at having to get involved
  - feeling unsure of what to take in.

Step 5: massaging the oesophagus reflexes
- massage the reflexes either with the thumbs or second fingers, with the caterpillar or rotation movement (pages 38–9)
- firmly but gently milk (pages 40–1) a few times with the thumbs
- lightly feather stroke (pages 41–2) with the second fingers.

Massaging the oesophagus reflexes:

- facilitates the ability to swallow life's experiences
- smoothes the progress of life's events
- creates an awareness of beneficial intake
- encourages an acceptance of nutritional values.

Airway reflexes

The airway reflexes (Figure 67), extend halfway along the inner edges of the balls of the feet from the bases of the big toes. They partially overlap the oesophagus reflexes.

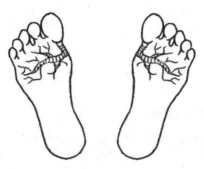

figure 67 airway reflexes

Massaging the airway reflexes:

- enhances the exchange of vital life-forces
- opens one up to all possibilities.

Elbow reflexes

The elbows reflexes are two protruding bones, midway down the outer edges of both feet (Figure 68).

The elbows provide 'elbow room' when needing space to be oneself.

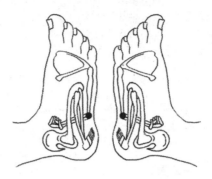

figure 68 elbow reflexes

Step 6: massaging the elbow reflexes
- place the thumbs or second fingers on these reflexes
- generously rotate (pages 38–9) to massage thoroughly
- firmly milk (pages 40–1) with the thumbs
- lightly feather stroke (pages 41–2) with the second fingers.

Massaging the elbow reflexes:

- makes room for each individual to just be!

Knee reflexes

The primary reflexes for the knees are situated in the centre of the balls of both feet, over the nipple reflexes (Figure 69) and the secondary reflexes are found on the outer edges of the feet, between the shoulder and elbow reflexes (Figure 70).

Knees allow the body and mind to bend and suddenly change direction with ease for greater progress to be made.

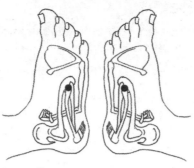

figure 69 primary knee reflexes

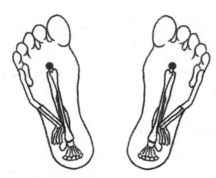

figure 70 secondary knee reflexes

Step 7: massaging the knee reflexes

- the primary reflexes are massaged with the breast reflexes (pages 121–2)
- to locate the secondary knee reflexes (Figure 71) place the thumbs on the shoulder reflexes and the third fingers on the elbow reflexes
- then use the second fingers to feel for the bony ledges, just above the midway point between the two digits
- replace the second fingers with the thumbs, apply slight pressure, release and massage thoroughly with a rotation movement (pages 38–9).

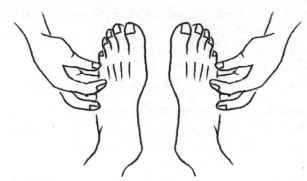

figure 71 locating the secondary knee reflexes

Massaging the knee reflexes:

- increases inner strength to move ahead
- enhances flexibility
- assists one in adapting to unexpected changes of direction more easily.

Solar plexus reflexes

The solar plexus reflexes (Figure 72) extend from the inner edges of both insteps, along the bases of the balls of both feet to the hollows at their centres. They are mainly accessed through the middle indentations.

The solar plexus are the most powerful reflexes on the feet since they are the 'abdominal brain' and are favourably or adversely affected by profound feelings about what is going on or not going on, hence the term 'having a gut feeling'.

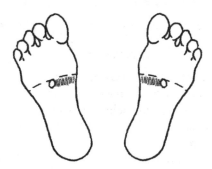

figure 72 solar plexus reflexes

The solar plexus reflexes are immediately affected by too much or too little emotion. They:

- sink when emotionally drained
- swell when overcome with emotion
- carry the lines and marks of inner turmoil and division.

Step 8: massaging the solar plexus reflexes
- place both thumbs on the hollows (Figure 73)
- apply gentle pressure until a slight resistance is felt
- keep the thumbs still for a while
- slowly ease the pressure until the tips of the thumbs are barely touching
- allow the thumbs to hover above the skin's surface for as long as necessary
- lightly stroke the reflexes
- remove the thumbs and lightly replace with the tips of the third fingers
- rest the finger tips on the hollows for a few seconds.

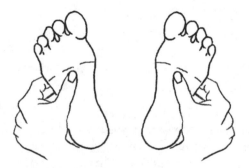

figure 73 massaging the solar plexus reflexes

Massaging the solar plexus reflexes:

- immediately calms mind, body and soul
- eases anxiety and panic attacks
- relieves asthmatic and bronchial spasms
- calms palpitations
- reduces hysteria
- regulates hyperventilation
- evokes incredible serenity and peace throughout.

Rib reflexes

The reflexes for the ribcage are on the sides and tops of both feet, mainly over the balls of the feet (Figure 74).

The ribcage emotionally reinforces and backs the whole, which is affected by all that is 'going on behind one's back' and all the emotional issues 'that have been put behind one'.

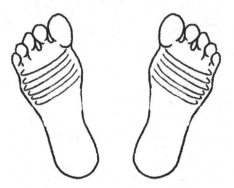

figure 74 ribcage reflexes

It reacts to 'getting it in the ribs' or when there is a 'thorn in one's side'.

Other forms of distress are reflected in the following ways.

The tops of the feet become:

- taut with strained ligaments when:
  - feeling under emotional pressure
  - seeking extra emotional backing and strength
  - trying to prop oneself up in an emotionally fraught environment
- puffy due to the presence of unshed tears.

Step 9: massaging the ribcage reflexes
- place the fingers either side of the balls of the feet and 'walk' them in unison over the tops of the feet (Figure 75)
- repeat several times
- use the heels of the hands to stroke the surfaces from the toes to the ankles
- lightly run all fingers in the same way.

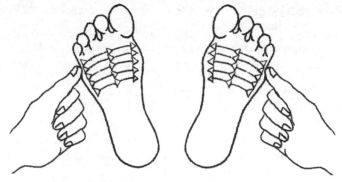

figure 75 massaging the ribcage reflexes

Massaging the ribcage reflexes:

- provides the inner strength to emotionally back oneself
- allows unresolved feelings to be resolved and dissipate.

Upper back reflexes

The upper thoracic vertebrae are reflected along both bony ridges on the inside edges of the balls of both feet (Figure 76).

The upper spine reflexes reflect the amount of emotional support that is perceivably available.

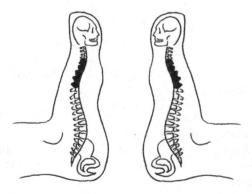

figure 76 upper back reflexes

When under pressure or during times of emotional distress, these bony ridges:

- collapse when there is little or no emotional support
- bulge to reach out for extra strength and emotional backing.

Step 10: massaging the upper back reflexes

- place the thumbs or second fingers on the ridge of bone immediately below the necks of the big toes (Figure 77)
- massage several times along the bony inside edges of the balls of the feet with either the caterpillar (pages 39–40) or rotation movements (pages 38–9)
- redo and alter the angle of the digit, first by gently pressing down on the reflexes to access the sensory nerve reflexes, and then repeat again by lightly pressing up against the reflexes to massage with the motor nerves
- milk (pages 40–1) with the thumbs
- feather stroke (pages 41–2) with the second fingers.

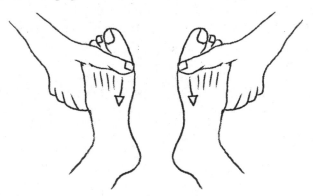

figure 77 massaging the upper back reflexes

Massaging the upper back reflexes:

- boosts emotional support
- provides inner strength.

The influence of reflexology on respiration and circulation

Massaging the balls of the feet liberates the breath. It eases tension in the rib cage so that the lungs can fully expand. In so doing latent contents of emotional congestion are subconsciously unravelled and released, thereby eliminating feelings of frustration, bewilderment and fear. This takes an enormous weight off the chest. The resultant sense of relief can be overwhelming and extremely invigorating.

Reflexology assists in the following ways:

- provides space to breathe
- gives an opportunity to get emotions off the chest
- boosts feelings of self-worth
- supports the nurturing process.

In between each sequence

Stroke both feet a few times, from the toes to the ankles (pages 41–2) and then move on to the massage of the insteps (page 137).

> If we wish for kindness,
> We need to be kind to ourselves,
> If we yearn for the truth,
> We need to be true to ourselves,
> For what we give of ourselves,
> Is always reflected back

10

the insteps

The insteps mirror the:

- liver
- pancreas
- spleen
- adrenal glands
- stomach
- duodenum
- jejunum
- small intestines
- large colon
- kidneys
- ovaries.

They reflect:

- actions
- reactions
- relationships
- communications.

The reflexes are related to the:

- third and fourth toes
- third and fourth fingers
- cheeks
- ears
- nose
- mouth
- lower arms
- shins
- wrists
- ankles.

The associated systems are:

- mainly digestive tract and its related organs
- part of the excretory system
- some of the reproductive systems.

Specific characteristics:

- represent fire and water
- resonate to yellow and orange.

The insteps reflect the following:

- the upper half of the right instep reflects the effect of all that was done or not done in the past
- the upper part of the left instep reveals present pursuits and one's ability to deal with current situations
- the lower half of the right instep shows the impact of previous relationships
- the left lower instep mirrors the state of on-going communications.

Natural characteristics of the insteps

The soft insteps are naturally flesh-coloured, vibrant, flexible areas, in the central part of the soles on both feet.

Impact of tension on the digestive process

The digestive process is immediately affected by a change of mind and a change of heart, as well as by fluctuating emotions that arise from extreme ecstasy to anger, fear, excitement, nervousness and insecurity regarding everything that is done or not done.

Detrimental reactions cause tension, which can:

- upset the harmonious expansion and contraction of the alimentary canal
- hamper the progress of food
- cause irritability
- increase acidity
- detrimentally alter the chemical composition of digestive juices and enzymes
- result in an excess covering of fat, which acts as a shock absorber against perceived outside attack.

Altered states of the insteps

Since the insteps mirror all that is going on or not going on in life, especially within personal relationships, their characteristics can regularly change due to a constant change of mind.

They can:

- become sunken
  - when drained and exhausted
- become swollen
  - when weighed down, burdened, overcome by the enormity of life's circumstances
- wrinkle the upper insteps
  - when concerned about actions
- wrinkle the lower insteps
  - when worried about relationships
- show crossed lines
  - when at a crossroads, angry or having a cross to bear
- display netted lines
  - when feeling entrapped and caught up
- have deep vertical lines
  - when divided as to what to do or how to relate.
- be covered with irregular, scattered lines
  - during periods of havoc and confusion.

The colours (pages 71–2) of the insteps demonstrate mood fluctuations regarding personal activities and relationships, whilst other significant markings can provide useful insight regarding the direction required for inner satisfaction and fulfilment.

Digestive, adrenal and kidney dis-orders relieved by reflexology

Regardless of the dis-order, a complete reflexology massage is always required, with specific attention to the:

- nervous system and solar plexus reflexes to calm the mind and relieve any pain, anxiety and fear
- endocrine gland reflexes to soothe the emotions and create inner harmony
- affected gland or organ reflexes to relax the distressed area and ease the symptoms of distress.

Reflexology assists specific ailments in the following ways:

- abdominal cramps: eases the gripping fear and anxiety about what to do or not do
- addictions: eliminates the need for self-destructive behavioural patterns by boosting one's self image.

- Addison's disease: provides fortification through an appreciation of one's own personal assets.
- adrenal disorders: boosts inner strength through greater understanding of one's self-worth.
- alcoholism: removes the need to drown one's sorrows through acceptance of oneself regardless of other's opinions
- anorexia: bolsters concepts of the self by providing a reason to exist
- appendicitis: replaces the fear and frustration of past communications with understanding and empathy
- appetite: provides a natural need for on-going sustenance
- belching: calms inner panic
- bowel disorders: eliminates wasted ideas and emotions that threaten present relationships and personal security releasing individuals from the perceived pressure of having to be a high achiever
- bulimia: provides the courage to take in life and do all that is required without feeling overwhelmed, threatened or inadequate
- cellulite: dismisses perceived obstructions and blockages by reinstating a belief in one's personal abilities
- cholelithiasis (inflammation of the gall bladder): replaces the bitterness and resentment of past actions with understanding and self forgiveness
- colic: pacifies maternal irritability, intolerance and impatience
- colitis: soothes fury at being hassled and put under constant pressure
- colon disorders: facilitates the expulsion of the remnants of life by replacing the dread of failure with self acceptance and recognition
- constipation: encourages the release of burdensome belief systems that threaten personal security
- diabetes: puts past unhappiness into perspective and brings back the joy and pleasure of being involved
- diarrhoea: eliminates the need to run away when feeling fearful or rejected
- haemorrhoids: removes the discontent of being encumbered, strained or suppressed
- hypoglycaemia: re-energizes the whole with renewed enthusiasm for the enjoyment of life

- liver disorders: dismisses inner fury, profound dissatisfaction and suppressed guilt and removes the need to be aggressive and continually critical of others
- malabsorption syndrome: replenishes mind, body and soul through an improved intake of the beneficial aspects of life
- middle back problems: releases guilt of all that 'one has turned one's back on' replacing it with the wisdom derived from life's experiences
- nephritis: eliminates anger and frustration at continual disappointments
- overweight: resolves weighty issues
- pancreatitis: ensures that all that is done is pleasurable
- peptic ulcer: stops the fear of inadequacy eating away at one by restoring belief in one's personal aptitude
- small intestine dis-orders: facilitates the absorption of the beneficial aspects of life
- solar plexus upsets: calms the 'abdominal brain' so that it is less sensitive and no longer overreacts to distressing, nerve-racking situations
- spastic colon: relieves the pressure and irritability of having to constantly meet self imposed expectations
- spleen disorders: reinstates balance, faith and appreciation in all activities
- starvation: replaces thoughts and feelings of deprivation and martyrdom with renewed self-worth
- stomach upsets: ensures inner tranquillity through the ability to manage new circumstances
- vomiting: encourages the acceptance of perceivably repulsive situations that are difficult to stomach through greater understanding.

Digestive reflexes

The upper and lower aspects of the digestive tract have their reflexes displayed on the sole insteps in the following way:

- the upper parts of the digestive tract are reflected onto the upper halves of the sole insteps, with those on the right foot displaying the impact of what was done or not done in the past and those on the left foot revealing how life situations are being dealt with or being left alone in the present

- the lower digestive organs are mirrored onto the lower halves of the sole insteps to display the effect of past relationships on the right foot and the impression of current communications on the left foot.

Liver reflexes

The liver is reflected through the triangular mound that occupies the bulk of the outer, upper quadrants of the right sole instep. A small portion is also reflected onto the left foot (Figure 78).

The liver is the largest and most versatile organ in the body and it performs a multitude of functions that keep mind, body and soul energized and active.

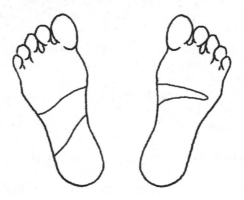

figure 78 liver reflexes

When frustrated or angry, especially about past actions and reactions or a lack thereof, the liver reflexes become:

- distended with excessive resentment
- sunken when exhausted from being pressurized into performing to meet social and family expectations.

Step 1: massaging the liver reflexes

- place the left thumb on the outer edge of the right foot, just below the instep, with the third finger directly opposite on top of the foot and the right thumb and third finger on the inner edge of the right foot, fractionally lower down
- either caterpillar (pages 39–40) or rotate (pages 38–9) the left thumb across the instep, with the third finger following as far as possible along the top

- finish above the right thumb
- remove the left digits
- massage in the opposite direction, from the inner to the outer edges with the right digits
- continue massaging back and forth across the liver reflex until the whole area has been covered
- milk (pages 40–1) firmly downwards, thumb over thumb
- feather-stroke (pages 41–2) lightly from top to bottom of the reflex with the third and fourth fingers
- the liver reflex on the left foot is massaged at the same time as the stomach reflex (pages 150–2).

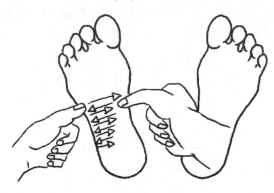

figure 79 massaging the liver reflexes

Massaging the liver reflexes keeps the liver in a harmonious state of well being so that it can effectively and efficiently:

- contribute abundant energy
- actively provide fuel for the physical expression and manifestation of ideas and feelings
- generate sufficient bodily heat for overall comfort
- detoxify and get rid of threatening elements
- modify chemical substances for beneficial usage based on past experiences
- act as a useful reservoir for blood.

Gall bladder reflexes

The gall bladder reflex is a tiny rounded swelling situated towards the centre of the right sole instep (Figure 80).

The gall bladder stores mainly broken down red blood cells, the nature of which is affected by memories of the amount of joy and pleasure derived from what was done or not done in the past. The greater the resentment the greater the bitterness within the bile.

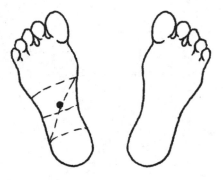

figure 80 gall bladder reflex

The gall bladder reflex hardens when there is accumulated bitterness at having to carry out particularly unpleasant or distasteful actions, e.g. during wars when forced to fight and kill generally against one's will. The memory of these atrocities often manifests in the next generation as gall stones.

Step 2: massaging the gall bladder reflex
- place the left thumb or third finger on the reflex and gently rotate (pages 38–9)
- milk (pages 40–1) downwards, thumb over thumb
- feather-stroke (pages 41–2) lightly with the third fingers.

Massaging the gall bladder reflex:

- assists in the efficient break down of worn out red blood cells
- facilitates the transportation of bile into the duodenum to assimilate fats for beneficial use
- prevents the accumulation of bitterness.

Pancreatic reflexes

The pancreatic reflexes, situated just above the 'waistline' of both feet, extend from the centres to the inner edges of each instep (Figure 81).

The pancreatic reflexes reveal the amount of satisfaction and pleasure being derived from personal pursuits and activities.

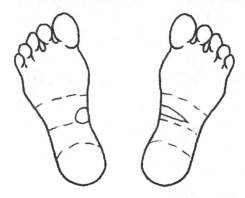

figure 81 pancreatic reflexes

Pancreatic disorders commonly occur 18 months to two years after a traumatic event that perceivably robs an individual of enjoying life to the full. As soon as the devastating event occurs, however, the pancreatic reflexes can provide vital clues of ways in which the spirit can replenish itself to prevent eventual disease.

The pancreatic reflexes:

- bulge to reach out for greater fulfilment
- become deflated when exhausted from trying to continually please others to the detriment of oneself.

Step 3: massaging the pancreatic reflexes

- place the left thumb across the left foot immediately below the waistline to use as a guideline (Figure 82)
- massage the left reflex with the right thumb, from right to left, several times either with the caterpillar (pages 39–40) or rotation (pages 38–9) movements
- milk (pages 40–1) also from right to left

- feather stroke (pages 41–2) downwards
- move the left thumb and place below the waistline on the right foot
- repeat the same procedure on the right reflex, as far as the centre, still progressing from right to left.

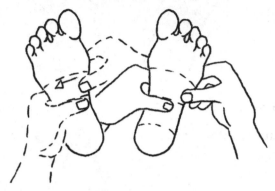

figure 82 massaging the pancreatic reflexes

Massaging the pancreatic reflexes:

- assists in maintaining a favourable sugary environment
- ensures the beneficial production of insulin and pancreatic juices
- helps to derive the greatest pleasure from all of life's events.

The spleen reflex

The reflex of the spleen is situated in the upper outer quadrant of the instep on the left foot (Figure 83).

The spleen ensures that all actions are accomplished with the appropriate amount of precision and attention to detail to ensure the most worthwhile and rewarding results.

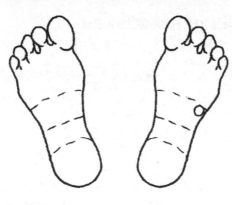

figure 83 the spleen reflex

The characteristics of this reflex change by:

- enlarging
  - with obsessive behaviour
  - when overwhelmed by the need for revenge, especially within the family
- sinking due to not being able to
  - stand up to strict rules
  - meet seemingly unrealistic and unreasonable expectations.

Step 4: massaging the spleen reflex
- place the thumbs either side of the reflex immediately below the balls of the left foot
- gently caterpillar (pages 39–40) or rotate (pages 38–9) the right thumb from right to left and the left thumb from left to right until the whole reflex has been thoroughly massaged
- milk (pages 40–1) firmly downwards, thumb over thumb
- feather stroke (pages 41–2) lightly with the third fingers.

Massaging the spleen reflex:

- encourages release from unreasonable pressure to perform
- balances one's approach to activities
- eases obsessions
- eliminates slovenliness
- makes activities worthwhile.

Adrenal gland reflexes

The adrenal reflexes are immediately below the solar plexus reflexes (pages 130–1), with the right reflex positioned slightly lower and more central than the left reflex (Figure 84).

The adrenal glands provide the courage and resourcefulness to put one's own unique and innovative ideas into practice regardless of any adversity that way-out, unusual concepts may initially evoke.

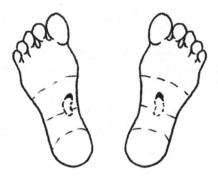

figure 84 adrenal gland reflexes

These reflexes swell when overwhelmed with fear, anxiety or terror and sink with defeatism, when lacking the courage of one's convictions or from being totally exhausted from continually having to prove oneself.

Step 5: massaging the adrenal gland reflexes
- place the thumbs or third fingers on the adrenal gland reflexes (Figure 84) with the right digit further in and fractionally more down than the left digit
- apply slight pressure and hold for a while
- very slowly release
- massage with gentle rotation movements (pages 38–9)
- lightly milk (pages 40–1) with the thumbs
- feather stroke (pages 41–2) with the third fingers
- finally rest the tips of the third fingers on the reflexes for a few seconds
- visualizing yellow enhances the effect.

Massaging the adrenal gland reflexes:

- puts mind, body and soul at ease by responding appropriately to real, rather than imagined, emergencies
- provides inner strength to achieve one's soul mission despite perceivable opposition
- makes the seemingly impossible possible.

Digestive reflexes

The bulk of the digestive organ reflexes are reflected onto the sole insteps.

The reflexology massage of the digestive tract, however, begins at the mouth reflexes in the big toes and ends in the anal reflexes on the inner heels.

Step 1: massaging the mouth reflexes (see pages 87–8)
- place the thumbs or fourth fingers on the mouth reflexes, just below the joints on the big toes
- apply slight pressure and gently rotate (pages 38–9)

Massaging the mouth reflexes:

- facilitates the chewing process
- improves the sense of taste.

Step 2: Massaging the oesophagus reflexes (see pages 126–7)
- use the caterpillar (pages 39–40), or rotation technique to massage down the inner edges of the balls of both feet.

Massaging the oesophgus reflexes:

- facilitates swallowing
- soothes the peristaltic action.

Cardiac sphincter reflexes

The reflexes of the cardiac sphincter are slight swellings, on the inner edges of both feet, situated where the balls of the feet and insteps meet (Figure 85).

The cardiac sphincter, the muscular entrance to the stomach, is immediately affected by overwhelming emotions, which either make it contract, causing nausea or vomiting, or expand, resulting in reflux and heart burn.

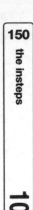
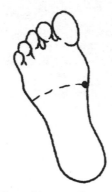
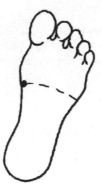

figure 85 cardiac sphincter reflexes

Step 3: massaging the cardiac sphincter reflexes
- rest the thumbs or second fingers on the reflexes
- apply slight pressure and hold for a few seconds
- slowly release
- lightly massage with a rotation movement (pages 38–9)
- gently stroke with the thumbs
- give extra attention for heartburn and hiatus hernia.

Massaging the cardiac sphincter reflexes:

- encourages receptivity of all life's events
- remains open to a variety of options.

Stomach reflexes

The stomach reflexes cover the bulk of the upper inner quadrant of the left instep, and part of the corresponding area on the right instep (Figure 86).

The stomach takes in food, breaks it down and alters it for digestion, all of which is symbolic of the way life is 'stomached' and dealt with.

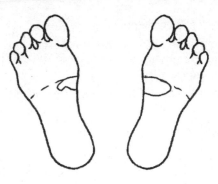

figure 86 stomach reflexes

The stomach is upset by unexpected actions, reactions and inactivity which manifest as:

- deep dread
- extreme concern
- fear of taking on anything new or unusual
- an inability to cope.

Step 4: massaging the stomach reflexes
- visualize the stomach reflex on the left foot (Figure 87)
- thoroughly massage either with the caterpillar (pages 39–40) or rotation technique (pages 38–9) from left to right with the left thumb
- then right to left with the right thumb
- milk (pages 40–1) in both directions and then only from right to left with both thumbs
- feather stroke (pages 41–2) with the third fingers
- repeat on the small stomach reflex on the right foot.

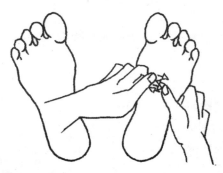

figure 87 massaging the stomach reflexes

Massaging the stomach reflexes:

- assists in stomaching life's experiences
- efficiently breaks down and transforms food into acceptable nutritional components
- enhances the ability to cope with current situations.

Pyloric sphincter reflex

The pyloric sphincter reflex is a slight swelling, on the right foot only, beneath the join of the second and big toe, where the balls of the feet and insteps meet (Figure 88).

The pyloric sphincter is the muscular outlet of the stomach, which is greatly influenced by the ability to process all that is being stomached or not stomached based on past memories. Fear causes it to contract, causing pyloric stenosis, which is more common in babies, especially males. It is linked to the mother's anxiety of having to deal with previous male issues.

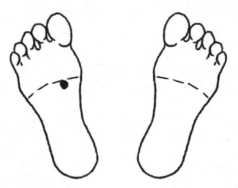

figure 88 pyloric sphincter reflex

Step 5: massaging the pyloric sphincter reflex
- rest the right thumb or third finger on the reflex
- apply slight pressure and hold for a few seconds
- slowly release
- lightly massage and then gently stroke.

Massaging the pyloric sphincter reflex:

- assists in deciding the best time to move onto the next stage.

Duodenum reflex

The duodenum reflex is C-shaped and follows the perimeter of the upper inner quadrant of the right sole instep (Figure 89).

The duodenum converts incoming nutritional substances, which represent daily events, into useful by-products, according to the way in which previous activities were taken in and dealt with or, in some situations, left untouched.

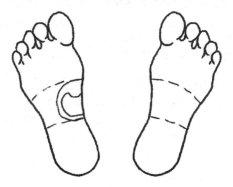

figure 89 duodenum reflex

Step 6: massaging the duodenum reflex

- continue from the pyloric sphincter reflex with the right thumb
- massage in a C-shaped movement either using the caterpillar (pages 39–40) or rotation (pages 38–9) movements
- change from the right to the left thumb midway to make the movement easier
- lightly milk (pages 40–1) then gently feather stroke (pages 41–2).

Massaging the duodenum reflex:

- encourages the effortless movement of on-going situations so that the greatest benefit can be derived from all past experiences
- ensures that only the best is taken out of each situation.

The jejunum reflex

The jejunum reflex extends along, or just above, the waistline from the end of the duodenum reflex to the beginning of the small intestine reflexes on the left foot (Figure 90).

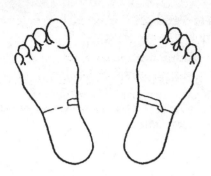

figure 90 jejunum reflex

Step 7: massaging the jejunum reflex

- massage several times from left to right with the left thumb
- lightly milk (pages 40–1), then gently feather stroke (pages 41–2).

Massaging the jejunum reflex:

- assists with moving onto the next stage, having dealt with past situations which helps in deciding what to take on and what to leave alone.

Small intestine reflexes

The small intestine reflexes occupy the lower halves of both insteps (Figure 91).

The small intestines take out of daily events those aspects of life that are beneficial for one's personal wellbeing. This is manifested through the absorption of favourable nutrients that energize the whole for personal growth within one's relationships, as well as in the development of new bodily cells.

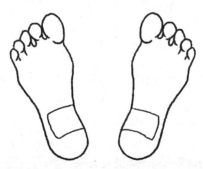

figure 91 small intestine reflexes

These reflexes are immediately affected by the give and take within individual interactions. They:

- swell when too much is being taken on
- flatten when excessively fearful or lacking in self-worth
- become deprived of vibrancy when exhausted
- dry up when drained from others constantly drawing on one's energy
- become lined when divided
- wrinkle when concerned or worried
- contain images to provide clues as to the next step.

Step 8: massaging the small intestine reflexes

- place the right thumb or fourth finger at the start of the small intestine reflex on the outer edge of the left foot (Figure 92)
- massage with the caterpillar (pages 39–40 or rotation movement (pages 38–9) along the waistline from right to left
- take the right thumb over to the right foot and continue massaging along the waistline of the right foot to the outer edge
- place the left thumb or fourth finger immediately below the right digit and massage the next strip from left to right on the right foot and then continue on the left foot
- at the outer edge on the left foot place the right thumb immediately below the left digit and massage from right to left continuing on the right foot
- continue this zig-zag movement until both lower insteps have been thoroughly massaged
- lightly milk (pages 40–1) with the thumbs
- gently feather stroke (pages 41–2) with the fourth fingers.

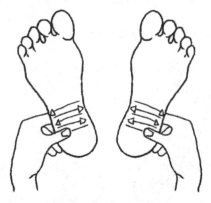

figure 92 massaging the small intestine reflexes

Massaging the small intestine reflexes:

- ensures the efficient absorption of nutrients
- creates greater tolerance within relationships
- balances give and take
- facilitates communications.

Ileo-caecal valve reflex

The ileo-caecal valve is situated towards the outer corner of the right lower instep (Figure 93).

The ileo-caecal valve is the muscular connection between the small and large intestines, which facilitates the onward movement of waste products. This is a very important reflex, especially for those hanging onto the past in one form or another.

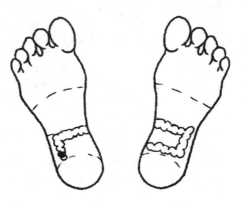

figure 93 ileo-caecal valve reflexes

Step 9: massaging the ileo-caecal valve reflex
- place the right thumb or fourth finger onto the reflex
- apply slight pressure and hold for a while
- very slowly release
- massage with gentle rotation movements (pages 38–9)
- lightly stroke
- finally rest the fourth fingers on the reflexes for a few seconds.

Massaging the ileo-caecal valve reflex:

• encourages the release of the old to make way for the new.

Appendix reflex

The appendix is reflected immediately below the ileo-caecal valve reflex in the lower outer corner of the right instep (Figure 94).

The appendix is surplus to body requirements and only plays a role in showing that certain relationships have come to a dead end.

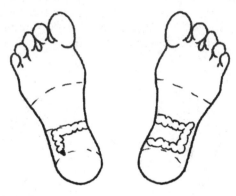

figure 94 appendix reflex

Step 10: massaging the appendix reflex
• place the left thumb or fourth finger at the base of the reflex (Figure 94)
• massage up the miniscule reflex with tiny rotation movements (pages 38–9)
• lightly stroke.

Large intestine reflexes

The large intestine, otherwise known as the colon, borders the lower halves of both sole insteps. It has four main sections (Figure 95):

• the ascending colon is reflected along the outer edge of the lower half of the right sole instep, next to the harder outer edge

- the transverse colon reflexes stretch across, or are fractionally below, the waistlines of both insteps
- the descending colon reflex extends down the outer edge of the lower half of the left sole instep, alongside the thick outer edge
- the sigmoid colon reflex, only on the left foot, follows the boundary between the instep and left heel.

The large intestine or colon contains remnants of the past. These wasted substances hold memories of what was not done and those things that were believed to be a complete waste of time. The colon itself mirrors the innate need for recognition of one's personal abilities.

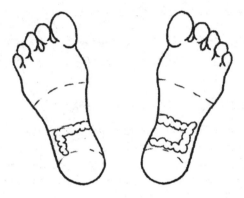

figure 95 large intestine/colon reflexes

The transverse colon reflexes, in particular, swell when individuals constantly compete against themselves and others or pressurize themselves to perform better than their personal best.

Ascending colon reflex

Step 11: massaging the ascending colon reflex
- place the left thumb or fourth finger on the lower, left corner of the right instep with the digit pointing upwards (Figure 96)
- massage upwards, along the reflex, as far as the waistline
- milk (pages 40–1) firmly with both thumbs
- feather stroke (pages 41–2) lightly with the fourth fingers.

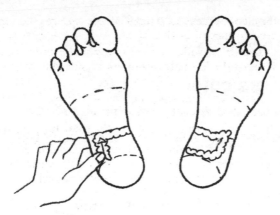

figure 96 massaging the ascending colon reflexes

Massaging the ascending colon reflexes:

- facilitates the on-going movement of life's remnants.

The hepatic flexure reflex

Step 12: massaging the hepatic flexure reflex
- feel for a swelling on or just below the waistline (Figure 97)
- apply slight pressure, hold for a while and then release
- turn the digit so that it is pointing towards the left foot.

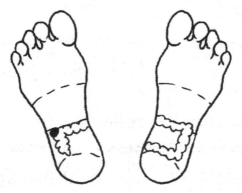

figure 97 hepatic flexure reflex

Massaging the hepatic flexure reflex:

- assists in turning corners.

Transverse colon reflexes

Step 13: massaging the transverse colon reflexes

- massage from left to right, with gentle rotation movements (pages 38–9), across the waistline of the right foot and then of the left foot (Figure 98)
- towards the centre of the left instep angle the thumb slightly upwards
- milk (pages 40–1) firmly with both thumbs
- feather stroke (pages 41–2) lightly with the fourth fingers.

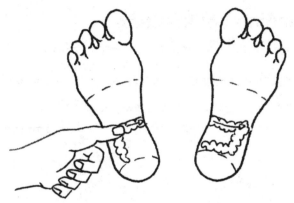

figure 98 massaging the transverse colon reflexes

Massaging the transverse colon reflexes:

- relieves one of the pressure of having to meet ridiculously high expectations.

Splenic flexure reflex

Step 14: massaging the splenic flexure reflex

- with your left thumb feel for the slight swelling of the splenic flexure reflex (Figure 99) fractionally up the outer upper corner of the left instep
- replace your left thumb with your right thumb angled downwards
- apply slight pressure, hold for a while and then release.

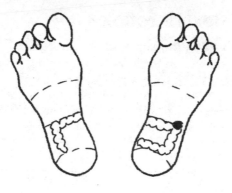

figure 99 splenic flexure reflex

Descending colon reflex

Step 15: massaging the descending colon reflex
- with the right thumb pointing downwards massage down the border of the outer edge of the left instep as far as the heel (Figure 100)
- milk (pages 40–1) firmly with both thumbs
- feather stroke (pages 41–2) lightly with the fourth fingers.

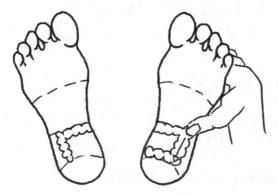

figure 100 massaging the descending colon reflex

Massaging the descending colon reflex:

- assists in letting go of irrational restraints and frustrating restrictions.

Sigmoid flexure reflex

Step 16: massaging the sigmoid flexure reflex

- rest the right thumb in the lower corner of the left sole instep (Figure 101)
- apply slight pressure, hold for a while and then release
- turn the thumb so that it is pointing towards the inside edge of the left foot.

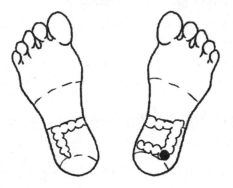

figure 101 sigmoid flexure reflex

Sigmoid colon reflex

Step 17: massaging the sigmoid colon reflex

- massage from right to left immediately above the left heel (Figure 102)
- milk (pages 40–1) firmly with both thumbs
- feather stroke (pages 41–2) lightly with the fourth fingers.

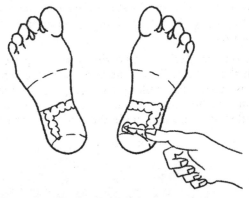

figure 102 massaging the sigmoid colon reflex

Massaging the sigmoid colon reflex:

- removes perceived obstructions that would otherwise prevent one from moving on
- encourages the on-going movement of remnants that are no longer of use.

Rectum and anal reflexes

The final release is through the rectum and anus, the reflexes of which are on the heels of both feet.

Step 18: massaging the rectum and anus reflexes

- massage these arcs well to complete the digestive process.

Upper female reproductive organ reflexes

Some female reproductive organs are reflected onto the soles, as well as the heels revealing ways in which feminine attributes can be used to enhance personal relationships.

Massaging these reflexes creates greater acceptance and appreciation of the female role in the formation, accommodation and nurturing of new beginnings.

Ovaries reflexes

The ovaries reflexes are situated in the outer lower corner of both insteps (Figure 103).

Ovaries reflect the ability to create and generate new concepts, not just in the form of babies, but also in shaping and developing on-going ideas.

The ovaries reflexes feel like two tiny water bubbles situated just beneath the surface. When menstruating, the reflex of the ovum that is about to ovulate enlarges, whilst that of the resting ovum virtually disappears. Since the contraceptive pill prevents ovulation it too can make these minute reflexes barely discernable.

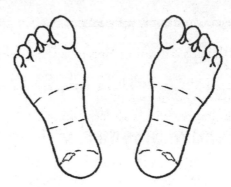

figure 103 ovaries reflexes

These reflexes swell when bursting with novel notions yet have no perceivable outlet. Alternatively they sink when amazing concepts are ignored by others, especially due to coming from a woman.

Step 1: massaging the ovaries reflexes
- massage these reflexes on both males and females because everybody has dual energies to varying degrees
- place the thumbs or fourth fingers on the ovaries reflexes (Figure 103) on both feet
- apply slight pressure and hold for a while
- very slowly release
- massage with gentle rotation movements (pages 38–9)
- lightly stroke
- then rest the fourth fingers on the reflexes for a few seconds
- visualizing orange enhances the effect.

Massaging the ovarian reflexes:

- encourages the generation of new concepts
- allows individuals to connect with their gentle and more sensitive feminine energies.

Fallopian tubes reflexes

The primary fallopian tubes and their finger reflexes stretch across both feet, between the instep and heels (Figure 104). Their secondary reflexes extend along the ankle creases on top of both feet (Figure 105).

Step 2: massaging the primary fallopian tube and finger reflexes

- place the thumbs or fourth fingers on the ovary reflexes (Figure 104)
- massage from the outer to the inner aspects with gentle rotation movements (pages 38–9)
- lightly milk (pages 40–1) with the thumbs
- then gently feather stroke (pages 41–2) with the fourth fingers.

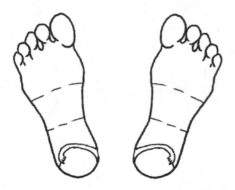

figure 104 primary fallopian tube and finger reflexes

Step 2: massaging the secondary fallopian tube and finger reflexes

- repeat the above on the secondary reflexes along the ankle creases (Figure 105).

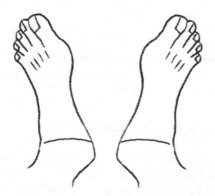

figure 105 secondary fallopian tube and finger reflexes

Uterus reflexes

The uterus reflexes are on the lower inside edges of both insteps (Figure 106).

The uterus or womb reflects the home, since it is the place of dwelling from conception until birth.

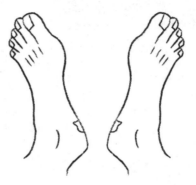

figure 106 uterus reflexes

These reflexes reflect the female principle and all that is happening or not happening within the home environment. The reflexes:

- look bruised when hurt at being taken advantage of or not receiving recognition because of being a women
- have small broken blood vessels due to intense unhappiness from perceived mental, emotional, physical or spiritual gender abuse
- swell when pregnant or making room for new concepts
- turn red when disappointed or frustrated at creativity not being accepted or recognized
- appear battered when unable to get ahead in a male dominated society
- develop a cut when home ties have been perceivably severed; it can also indicate a hysterectomy in females.

Step 3: massaging the uterus reflexes

- gently massage these reflexes (Figure 106) either with a caterpillar (pages 39–40 or rotation (pages 38–9) movement
- lightly milk (pages 40–1) with the thumbs
- fleetingly feather stroke (pages 41–2) with the fourth fingers especially during pregnancy.

Massaging the uterus reflexes:

- creates a more harmonious environment within the home
- balances feminine energy.

Pregnant reflexes

During pregnancy these reflexes enlarge or develop a shadow in the shape of the developing embryo:

- around six weeks after conception an embryonic shape can usually be detected in the uterine reflex on the inside of one or occasionally both feet (Figure 107)
- in 90% of pregnancies the baby is a boy if the swelling is on the right instep, which reflects masculine energies, and a girl if on the left foot, where female energies are more evident.

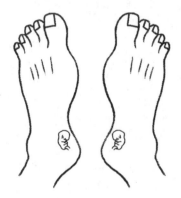

figure 107 around six weeks of pregnancy

- when the developing foetus becomes more noticeable in the mother-to-be's body, the foetal reflexes become increasing obvious on the corresponding parts of the feet (Figure 108)
- due to the accuracy of the reflection it is possible to determine the various body parts of the unborn baby, especially the head and buttocks, as well as its position in the womb
- as the foetus grows and develops in the body, its reflection expands accordingly on the feet.

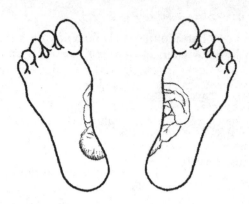

figure 108 reflection of the developing foetus

- when the baby's head engages in the pelvic cavity, a rounded swelling can often be seen on the edges of the heels of the feet, near the insteps (Figure 109)

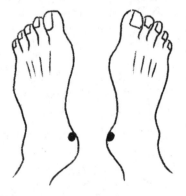

figure 109 engaged head of the developing foetus

Reflexology before, during and after pregnancy

Step 1: reflexology before conception

Both parents should receive reflexology on a regular basis, ideally for at least a year before the pregnancy.

For the father-to-be, this:

- ensures strong, healthy sperm
- prepares him physically, mentally, emotionally and spiritually
- provides the inner strength and intuition to support the mother-to-be during the pregnancy.

For the mother-to-be, this:

- ensures a healthy womb
- boosts inner resourcefulness
- raises consciousness
- increases intuitive awareness
- enhances receptiveness of the baby on all levels
- creates inner joy and peacefulness.

Step 2: reflexology during pregnancy

- both the mother-to-be and foetus thrive on reflexology
- father-to-be also needs on-going treatment so that he can tune into the mother-to-be's innate needs in a relaxed manner
- the reflexology touch should be gentle, light and loving, especially over the womb reflexes
- give extra attention to the breasts, uterus, pelvic and vaginal reflexes
- encouraging the father-to-be to give the reflexology to his partner is an ideal way of involving him.

Reflexology during pregnancy:

- ensures a relaxed, healthy atmosphere internally and externally
- eliminates the incidence of:
  - morning sickness due to the innate knowledge of being able to cope
  - back pain from becoming more capable of backing and supporting oneself
  - varicose veins by making the whole journey pleasurable
- enhances the blood flow to the womb
- maintains good provision of vital life-forces for the developing foetus
- keeps the mother well, happy and content.

If the baby is in a breach or unnatural position, rotate the little toes of the mother, to encourage it to turn.

Step 3: Reflexology during childbirth

Reflexology during childbirth is excellent, especially when administered by the father-to-be. It:

- calms and reassures the mother-to-be
- involves and occupies the father-to-be
- facilitates the process because body, mind and soul are relaxed
- encourages appropriate and beneficial involvement of the expectant mother and father
- makes the whole experience more enjoyable.

Even when the cervix is fully dilated, it has been found that the mother more readily participates in the childbirth process when her big toes draw back and all her little toes extend forwards (Figure 110).

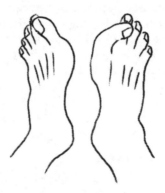

figure 110 mother ready for active participation in childbirth process

Step 4: reflexology after childbirth

If both parents continue to receive reflexology, they will be more relaxed and calm. The baby also loves its feet being massaged, especially during feeding. It:

- helps mind, body and soul to adapt to the new, exciting circumstance
- with calmer parents, the baby is able to relax and sleeps more soundly
- reduces anxiety and the incidence of vomiting, colic and other childhood dis-orders

- helps both parents cope with the unexpected
- maintains a loving, homely relationship.

Excretory reflexes

Also present in the instep area are some excretory reflexes. These reveal the ability to let go of unnecessary, time-consuming relationships.

Kidney reflexes

The kidney reflexes (Figure 111) are tiny vertical mounds situated beneath the adrenal gland reflexes (Figure 84). The right reflex is slightly lower and further in than the left.

The kidneys continually purify the blood and maintain a favourable water balance by filtering out worked through thoughts and emotions that are no longer of value to mind, body and soul.

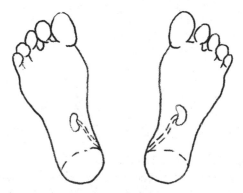

figure 111 kidney reflexes

The condition of these reflexes is influenced by the give and take in partnerships. The reflexes:

- swell with the enormity of taking on too much
- harden when disappointed or disillusioned
- sink when deflated or defeated.

Step 1: massaging the kidney reflexes
- place the thumbs or fourth fingers pointing downwards at the top of both reflexes (Figure 111)
- massage from top to bottom either with the caterpillar (pages 39–40) or rotation techniques (pages 38–9)
- milk (pages 40–1) thoroughly with the thumbs
- feather stroke (pages 41–2) with the third and fourth fingers.

Massaging the kidney reflexes:

- encourages the efficient filtering and purification of blood and its contents
- ensures a harmonious chemical environment
- maintains an ideal fluid balance
- assists in draining toxic substances that are detrimental to inner harmony.
- purifies mind, body and soul.

Ureter reflexes

The ureter reflexes (Figure 112) extend from the mid point of the kidney reflexes (Figure 111) to the swollen mounds at the bases of the insteps on the inner edges of both feet, which are the bladder reflexes (Figure 122).

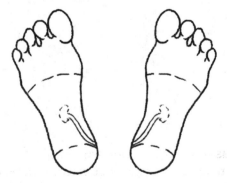

figure 112 ureter reflexes

Step 2: massaging the ureter reflexes
- place the thumbs or fourth fingers halfway down the kidney reflexes (Figure 112)

- massage either with the caterpillar (pages 39–40) or rotation techniques (pages 38–9) along these reflexes from the kidney to the bladder reflexes
- milk (pages 40–1) with the thumbs
- feather stroke (pages 41–2) with the fourth fingers.

Step 3: massaging the bladder (pages 185–6) and urethra reflexes (pages 186–7)

These reflexes are situated in the heel region and represent sufficient security within oneself to finally let go of worked through notions and beliefs.

Lower arm reflexes

The lower arms reflexes (Figure 113) extend from the protruding bones, midway along the outer edges of both feet, to the swellings beneath the outer ankle-bones.

The lower arms reach out to assist in the activities of life.

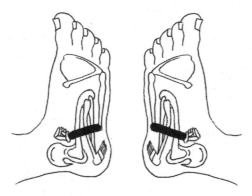

figure 113 lower arm reflexes

Step 1: massaging the lower arm reflexes
- use the thumbs or third fingers to massage these reflexes either with the caterpillar (pages 39–40) or rotation movement (pages 38–9)
- thoroughly milk (pages 40–1) with the thumbs
- gently feather stroke (pages 41–2) with the third fingers.

Massaging the lower arm reflexes:

- provides the expansiveness to embrace the enormity of all that needs to be dealt with on a daily basis.

Wrist reflexes

The wrist reflexes are immediately beneath the swelling under both outer ankle-bones (Figure 114).

The wrists provide the flexibility to handle the many differing aspects of life, especially when it comes to dealing with others.

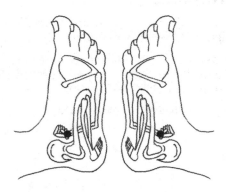

figure 114 wrist reflexes

Shin reflexes

The shin reflexes (Figure 115) extend from the knee reflexes (Figures 69–70) to the feet reflexes (Figures 129–30) on the outer edges of both feet.

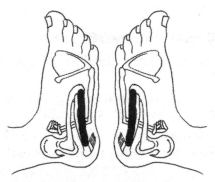

figure 115 shin reflexes

Step 2: massaging the shin reflexes

- use the thumbs or third fingers to massage these reflexes either with the caterpillar (pages 39–40) or rotation movement (pages 38–9)
- thoroughly milk (pages 40–1) with the thumbs
- gently feather stroke (pages 41–2) with the third fingers.

Massaging the shin reflexes provides the scope and strength to allow activities to progress.

Ankle reflexes

The ankle reflexes (Figure 116) are situated next to the feet reflexes (Figures 129–30) on the outer edges of both feet.

The ankles assist individuals in adapting to the ups and downs encountered on the journey through life, especially within one's communications and relationships.

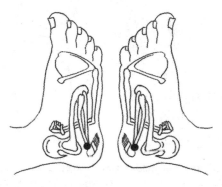

figure 116 ankle reflexes

Middle back reflexes

The middle back is reflected onto the tops of both feet, opposite the insteps (Figure 117).

The middle back reflexes reveal backing for all activities as well as within communications. They also mirror:

- perceived activities going on behind one's back
- all those things that one has turned one's back on.

Unnatural middle back reflexes include:

- the development of a prominent bone on top of the foot indicating that the individual is being pressurized into meeting high standards and/or unrealistic expectations
- veins appear over this area when unhappy about things that are happening or not happening being put in the background.

Step 1: massaging the middle back reflexes
- place all fingers on the outer edges of both feet (Figure 117)
- 'walk' the fingers in unison over the tops of both feet from the outer to the inner edges
- repeat several times
- then lightly run the tips of all fingers over the tops of both feet from the base of the toes to the ankle creases.

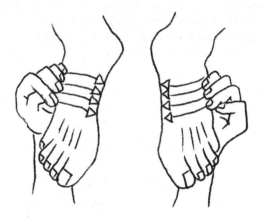

figure 117 massaging the middle back reflexes

Massaging the middle back reflexes provides the inner strength to carry on.

Lumber vertebrae reflexes

The lumber vertebrae reflexes extend along the central portion of the ridges of bone situated on the inner edges of both feet.

The lumber vertebrae reflexes show the amount of support that is perceivably being received for all that is done or not done, as well as backing within personal relationships.

The bones that make up these reflexes:

- bulge when reaching out for extra understanding and back-up
- sink when collapsing from the strain of having to support oneself and others, or when not receiving any perceivable backing.

Step 2: massaging the lumber vertebrae reflexes

- place the thumbs on the reflexes where the balls of the feet and insteps meet (Figure 118)
- massage either with the caterpillar (pages 39–40) or rotation movement (pages 38–9)
- repeat several times
- shift the position so that the thumbs press gently down onto the reflexes to massage the sensory nerves or push lightly upwards to massage the motor nerves
- thoroughly milk (pages 40–1) with the thumbs
- gently feather stroke (pages 41–2) with the third fingers.

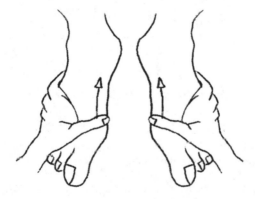

figure 118 massaging the lumber vertebrae reflexes

Massaging the lumber vertebrae reflexes:

- strengthens backing within all activities and relationships
- bolsters support for all that is done or not done
- backs up communications.

Internal abdominal organ reflexes

Step 3: massaging the internal abdominal organ reflexes

- place the thumbs or all fingers on the inner edges of the fleshy insteps, where the balls of the feet and insteps meet (Figure 119)
- massage using either the caterpillar (pages 39–40) or rotation movement (pages 38–9)
- thoroughly milk (pages 40–1) and gently feather stroke (pages 41–2).
- very lightly stroke both insteps with the backs of the hands.

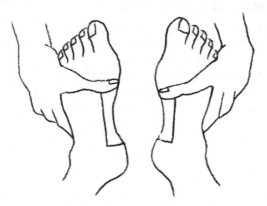

figure 119 massaging the internal abdominal organ reflexes

Massaging the internal abdominal organ reflexes:

- provides inner strength to put one's own ideas into practice
- encourages resourcefulness through the utilisation of personal skills
- provides an inner peace for the harmonious expansion and contraction of the alimentary canal.

Effect of reflexology on the digestive process

Reflexology calms the digestive process and makes it easier to deal with daily events and cope with all that is on one's plate in the following ways:

- everything becomes more palatable through improved taste
- makes it effortless to chew over challenging dilemmas

- delicious to swallow
- pleasant to stomach
- agreeable to absorb
- gratifying to let go of the wasteful and time-consuming aspects of life.

In time, massaging the feet takes a weight off the mind and body, replacing it with a healthy intake and hearty appetite for life, accompanied by renewed energy and the enthusiasm to enjoy it.

In between each sequence

Stroke both feet a few times, from the toes to the ankles (page 111) and then move onto the massage of the heels (pages 183–96).

> *Think only the best,*
> *Do only the best,*
> *Expect only the best.*

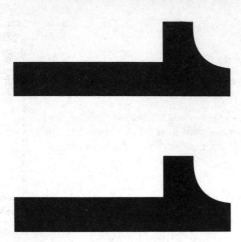

the heels

In this chapter you will find out:
- that your spiritual feet lead you within and your earthly feet keep you on track, without having to dig your heels in!

The heels mirror the:

- pelvic bones
- hands
- feet
- lower urinary system
- reproductive glands and organs
- lower back.

They reflect:

- basic security
- mobility
- stability
- personal growth
- individuality.

The reflexes are related to the:

- small toes
- little fingers
- jaw.

Associated body systems are:

- muscular
- skeletal
- excretory
- reproductive.

Specific characteristics:

- represent earth
- resonate to red and pink.

Natural characteristics of the heels

The heels are naturally flesh-coloured, rotund mounds.

Like firm, pliable cushions, the heels put a spring into the step and act as the shock absorbers of the body every time the foot is put down.

Altered states of the heels

Self-imposed limitations are immediately reflected onto the heels, which:

- become bruised when wounded at the direction of life or the lack of it
- become cracked when divided and pulled in many directions
- harden when difficulty in making progress
- develop tough rims when digging the heel in
- become heavy when life is heavy going
- are painful during perceivably unpleasant growing experiences
- roughen with a rough, challenging path
- become spongy when giving in too easily
- diminish in size from having to tread carefully, especially over egg shells.

The colour of the skin indicates the emotion involved (see pages 71–2).

Effect of tension

Limited social beliefs impose limitations and restraints that hamper personal progress, whilst self-doubt, uncertainty and fear stunt personal growth and development on all levels of mind, body and soul.

Reproductive, skeletal, muscular and urinary dis-orders relieved through reflexology

Regardless of the dis-order, a complete reflexology massage is always required, with specific attention to the:

- nervous system and solar plexus reflexes to calm the mind and relieve any pain, anxiety and fear
- endocrine gland reflexes to soothe the emotions and create inner harmony
- affected gland or organ reflexes to relax the distressed area and ease the symptoms of distress.

Reflexology assists specific ailments in the following ways:

- amenorrhoea: removes embarrassment or fear of being a female
- anal bleeding: lets go of all the sadness at the waste of time and energy
- anal disorders: eliminates the frustration at the lack of progress
- arms: strengthens the ability and capacity to embrace the fullness of life
- bed wetting: replaces insecurity and lack of control with an inner confidence
- birth defects: eliminates extreme anxiety and encourages the release of inherent belief system that are no longer applicable
- bone: bolsters inner strength and personal support
- broken or fractured bone: eases resistance to outside control and facilitates a break from limiting circumstances
- bone deformity: liberates the mind from the perceived pressures of having to bow and bend into unsuitable belief structures
- bursitis: soothes inflamed thoughts regarding sudden and unexpected changes in the direction of life's circumstances
- buttocks: assists in regaining power, security and basic support for life
- cystitis: expels the frustration and anger of feeling continually fed up from holding onto wasted emotions that threaten personal security
- lower back pain: dissipates the hurt at not feeling backed, especially financially, by enriching mind, body and soul.

Rectum reflexes

The rectum is reflected in the shape of an arc, on the inside surfaces of both feet (Figure 120).

These reflexes represent the relief of finally letting go of wasteful and rough substances from mind, body and soul.

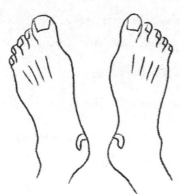

figure 120 rectum reflexes

Their appearance alters as they:

- swell from being constipated due to the fear of letting go
- sink from diarrhoea, when on the run
- turn red from haemorrhoids that develop when there is a fearful deadline
- look red and distended from diverticulitis indicating anger at not being able to find another outlet for wasteful circumstance or from constantly reaching a dead end.

Step 1: massaging the rectum reflexes

- place the thumbs or little fingers at the junction of the heel and instep, on the inner edges of both feet (Figure 120)
- massage the arched reflexes either with the caterpillar (pages 39–40) or rotation (pages 38–9) movements
- firmly milk (pages 40–1) and gently feather stroke (pages 41–2).

Massaging the rectum reflexes:

- facilitates the final release of wasteful substances
- eases constipation
- calms diarrhoea
- strengthens or relaxes the anal sphincters as required.

Anus reflexes

The anus reflexes are situated in indentations, midway between the inner ankle-bones and the tips of the inside heels (Figure 121).

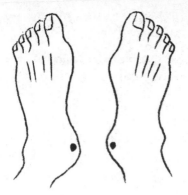

figure 121 anus reflexes

Step 2: massaging the anus reflexes
- rest the little fingers on the reflexes (Figure 121)
- apply slight pressure, hold for a few seconds and then release
- stroke with the thumbs.

Massaging the anus reflexes loosens the tight grip on the desperate need to be in control.

Bladder reflexes

The bladder reflexes are the fleshy mounds on the inside edges of both insteps at the junction with the heels (Figure 122).

The bladder acts as reservoir for worked through thoughts and emotions until mind, body and soul are ready to let go.

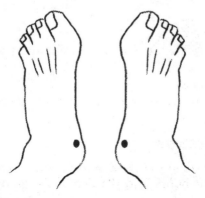

figure 122 bladder reflexes

These reflexes swell considerably when unhappy and 'pissed off' usually with the sexual partner.

Step 3: massaging the bladder reflexes

- place the thumbs or all fingers on the fleshy mounds on both feet (Figure 122)
- massage thoroughly either with the caterpillar (pages 39–40) or rotation techniques (pages 38–9)
- milk (pages 40–1) with the thumbs
- feather stroke (pages 41–2) with the little fingers.

Massaging the bladder reflexes:

- facilitates the release of discarded thoughts and emotions
- lets go of the need to constantly hang on.

Urethra reflexes

The urethra reflexes extend from the fleshy mounds, on the inner aspects of both feet to:

- the slight indentations, midway between the inner ankle bone and tip of the heel, on females (Figure 123)
- the heel tips on males (Figure 124).

The urethra has two muscular sphincters that control the release of urine from the body. This ability is temporarily lost when feeling fearful or insecure, especially in threatening situations that could usurp one's position and status in life, over which one has no control.

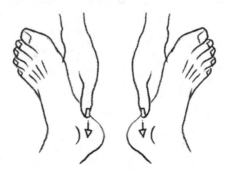

figure 123 massaging female urethra reflexes

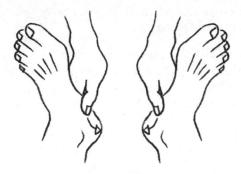

figure 124 massaging male urethra reflexes

Step 4: massaging the urethral reflexes
- place the thumbs or little fingers at the start of the reflexes on the edges of the fleshy mounds (Figures 123 and 124)
- massage along the reflexes either with the caterpillar (pages 39–40) or rotation techniques (pages 38–9)
- concentrate on the slight indentation on females and the tips of the heels on males
- milk (pages 40–1) with the thumbs
- feather stroke (pages 41–2) with the little fingers.

Massaging the urethral reflexes:

- strengthens or relaxes the sphincters as appropriate
- eases enuresis (bed wetting) and incontinence
- soothes the flow of urine
- creates inner control especially in frighful situations.

Pelvic bone reflexes

The pelvic bone reflexes occupy most of the heel pads and the surrounding areas (Figure 125).

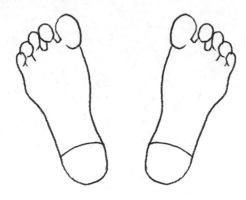

figure 125 pelvic bone reflexes

Step 5: massaging the pelvic reflexes
- place the thumbs or little fingers on the outer edges of both heel pads, at the junction with the insteps (Figure 125)
- gently massage in horizontal strips from the outer to the inner edges of the heels with either the caterpillar (pages 39–40) or rotation technique (pages 38–9)
- repeat by, placing the digit fractionally lower down the heels each time
- continue until both heel pads have been thoroughly massaged
- milk (pages 40–1) with the thumbs, in vertical strips downwards, from the outer to the inner edges
- lightly feather stroke (pages 41–2) with the little fingers, from top to bottom, finishing on the inner edges.

Massaging the pelvic reflexes:

- provides a solid foundation for self-development
- enhances flexibility and mobility
- facilitates childbirth.

Hip reflexes

The hips are reflected onto both outer ankle-bones, with the bony swellings beneath these reflecting the ball and socket joints at the tops of the legs (Figure 126).

The hips propel the body through life and provide the motivation and incentive to move ahead and get going.

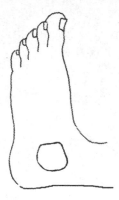

figure 126 hip reflexes

Step 6: massaging the hip reflexes
- massage around the outer ankle-bones either with the thumbs or all fingers using the caterpillar (pages 39–40) or rotation technique (pages 38–9)
- repeat several times
- milk (pages 40–1) thoroughly with the thumbs
- lightly feather stroke (pages 41–2) with the little fingers.

Massaging the hip reflexes provides the impetus and force to move ahead with ease.

Buttock reflexes

The buttock reflexes are on the rounded mounds beneath the outer ankle-bones on both feet (Figure 127).

The buttocks are the position of power and their reflexes reflect the amount of command one has over the direction in one's life. Flabby buttocks indicate being out of control and reliant on others for basic security, whilst exceptionally taut buttocks keep an extremely tight rein and a firm control on all affairs, especially the purse strings.

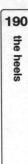

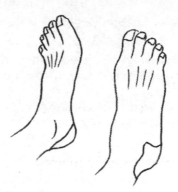

figure 127 buttock reflexes

Step 7: massaging the buttock reflexes

- massage the whole of the outer triangular areas of the heels either with the thumbs or all fingers using the caterpillar (pages 39–40) or rotation technique (pages 38–9)
- repeat several times
- milk (pages 40–1) thoroughly with the thumb
- lightly feather stroke (pages 41–2) with the little fingers.

Massaging the buttock reflexes empowers the individual.

Hand reflexes

The hand reflexes are the soft swellings, on top of both feet, in front of the outer ankle-bones (Figure 128).

Hands handle life, manipulate and mould on-going situations on a daily basis, whilst the fingers deal with the finer details of life.

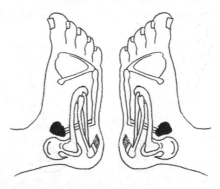

figure 128 hand reflexes

The characteristics of these reflexes change when pressurized. They:

- swell when there is an enormous amount that needs handling
- withdraw and sink when fearful or dubious about dealing with life events
- develop broken blood vessels indicating unhappiness at the way in which situations are being handled or not being dealt with.

Step 8: massaging the hand reflexes
- place the thumbs or all fingers on the fleshy mounds on both feet (Figure 128)
- massage thoroughly either with the caterpillar (pages 39–40) or rotation techniques (pages 38–9)
- milk (pages 40–1) with the thumbs
- feather stroke (pages 41–2) with the little fingers.

Massaging the hand reflexes facilitates the handling all of life's experiences.

Feet reflexes

The feet are reflected onto the central portion of the lower edges of both heel pads (Figure 129), as well as onto the outer surfaces, beneath the outer ankle bones (Figure 130).

Feet represent stability and security, as well as the ability to move ahead and make progress through life.

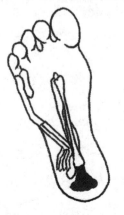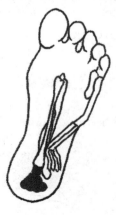

figure 129 feet reflexes on the heel pads

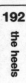

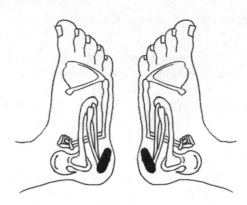

figure 130 feet reflexes on the outer edges

The foot reflexes bulge when life is perceived to be a drag or heavy going.

Step 9: massaging the feet reflexes
- massage all reflexes thoroughly with the rotation technique (pages 38–9)
- milk (pages 40–1) with the thumbs
- feather stroke (pages 41–2) with the little fingers.

Massaging the feet reflexes provides stability and mobility for personal security, growth and development.

Lower reproductive reflexes

The reflexes of the lower reproductive organs and glands are reflected onto the inner surfaces of both heels.

These reflexes represent male and female principles.

Vagina reflexes

The vagina is reflected onto the hollows between the inner ankle-bones and heel tips on the insides of both feet (Figure 131).

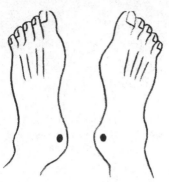

figure 131 vagina reflexes

The vagina reflexes expand when feeling overwhelmed at having to meet and fulfil unrealistic expectations because of being a woman, whilst broken blood vessels or bruising over these reflexes reflect perceived sexual abuse, either physical, mental or emotional.

Step 10: massaging the vaginal reflexes
- place the little fingers on these reflexes and gently rotate
- milk lightly (pages 40–1) with the thumbs
- soothingly feather stroke (pages 41–2) with the little fingers.

Massaging the vaginal reflexes encourages acceptance of one's feminity.

Male reproductive reflexes

The male reproductive organs and glands are situated on the inside of the heels on both feet (Figure 132).

The male reproductive organs reflect a man's perception of himself and his ease or dis-ease with his designated role in life. They function according to his ability to rise to the occasion and perform as a man. Impotence occurs when not feeling important or respected.

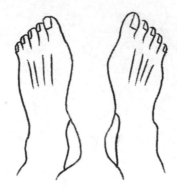

figure 132 male reproductive reflexes

Step 11: massaging the male reproductive reflexes

- massage the inner triangular areas of both heels either with the thumbs or all fingers using the caterpillar (pages 39–40) or rotation technique (pages 38–9)
- repeat several times
- milk (pages 40–1) thoroughly with the thumb
- lightly feather stroke (pages 41–2) with the little fingers.

Massaging the male reproductive reflexes:

- improves strength and performance
- makes one feel important
- encourages the individual to rise appropriately to any given occasion.

Testes reflexes

The testes are reflected anywhere between the hollows on the inner ankle-bones and the tips of the heels on the insides of both feet (Figure 133) because of their tendency to hang loose when hot and withdraw when cold.

The testes indicate the ability make an adequate contribution to society, with the sperm count being a direct reflection of this, as they test their way through life.

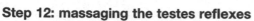

figure 133 testes reflexes

Step 12: massaging the testes reflexes
- place the little fingers on these reflexes (Figure 133) and gently rotate
- milk lightly (pages 40–1) with the thumbs
- soothingly feather stroke (pages 41–2) with the little fingers.

Massaging the testes reflexes ensures a worthwhile contribution to the development and progress of humanity.

Lower back reflexes

The coccyx and sacrum bones of the lower back are reflected at the base of the bony ridges along the inner insteps. The reflexes curve under the inner ankle-bones on both feet (Figure 134).

The lower back provides the perceived security and backing required to expand and explore new horizons.

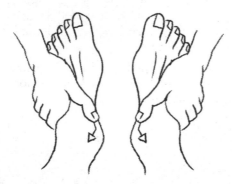

figure 134 massaging the lower back reflexes

These reflexes become distended when reaching out for greater financial backing and support and collapse when there are insufficient funds or where there is a drain on personal resources.

Step 13: massaging the lower back reflexes

- place the thumbs or all fingers on the bony ridges along the inner edges of both insteps, where the insteps and heels meet (Figure 134)
- massage well along the reflexes using either the caterpillar (pages 39–40) or rotation movement (pages 38–9)
- repeat several times
- milk well (pages 40–1) and lightly feather stroke (pages 41–2).

Massaging the lower back reflexes:

- eases lower back pain
- improves self-worth
- provides basic support and security
- encourages greater resourcefulness.

In between each sequence

Stroke both feet a few times, from the toes to the ankles (page 111) and then move onto the finale (pages 198–202).

Live your life as an exclamation, not as an explanation!

12

the finale

In this chapter you will
recognize:
- that health and healing are
  only two feet away!

The body, mind and soul should be completely relaxed by now, making it an ideal opportunity to gently stretch and extend the feet for greater flexibility and expansion of mind, body and soul.

Step 1: stretching the mind and spine
- gently pull both little toes simultaneously, then the fourth toes, followed by the third and second toes, and finally the two big toes
- pull the big toes for longer.

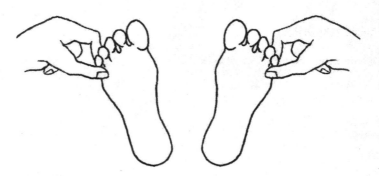

figure 135 stretching the mind and spine

Stretching the mind and spine provides tremendous relief for:

- neck tension
- headaches
- back disorders.

Step 2: extending the neck
- lightly support the base of the right little toe with the left thumb and index finger
- hold the right little toe between the right thumb and index finger
- rotate this little toe first anti-clockwise and then clockwise
- repeat on the fourth right toe then the rest of the toes on the right foot
- do the same on the left foot, starting with the left little toe and finishing with the left big toe
- spend time on rotating the big toes.

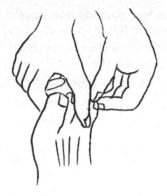

figure 136 extending the neck

Extending the neck:

- eases neck stiffness
- increases flexibility.

Step 3: flexing the upper body

- embrace the upper part of the right foot with the palms of the hands placed either side of both feet
- gently roll the foot from side to side by moving the hands alternately up and down
- repeat on the left foot.

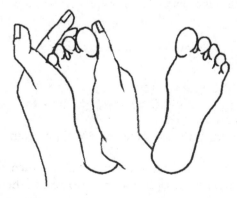

figure 137 flexing the upper body

Flexing the upper body:

- facilitates the give and take
- eases expansion and contraction
- boosts morale.

Step 4: expanding mind, body and soul
- place both hands on top of the feet
- gently but firmly stretch them downwards
- now place the palms of the hands flat against the soles of both feet and gradually ease them upwards.

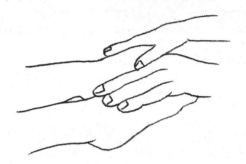

figure 138 expanding mind, body and soul

Expanding mind, body and soul:

- opens the whole to on-going opportunities
- broadens horizons.

Step 5: flexing the lower body
- support the right heel with the left hand
- use the right hand to rotate the right foot, first anti-clockwise and then clockwise
- change hands and repeat on the left foot.

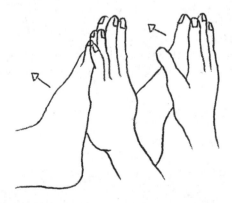

figure 139 flexing the lower body

Flexing the lower body:

- balances the odds
- keeps life events in proportion.

Step 6: loosening the whole

- place the thumbs beneath the right little toe necks with the fingers immediately opposite on top of the feet
- gently push the thumbs up whilst lightly stretching the tops of the feet outwards with the finger
- repeat this movement several times
- gradually progress down the length of the foot to the right ankle.
- repeat on the left foot.

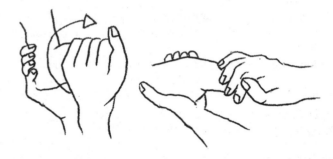

figure 140 loosening the whole

Loosening the whole:

- encourages a more relaxed and contented approach to life
- energizes the whole.

Step 7: final step

- complete the reflexology sequence by massaging the solar plexus reflexes (see pages 130–1) for about a minute.

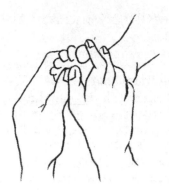

figure 141 final step

Step 8: ending the session

- stroke first the right foot from top to bottom and then the left foot
- cover both feet with the sheet or blanket
- continue holding the covered feet and in a soft voice invite the recipient to take in three deep breathes before opening their eyes
- allow them to surface in their own time
- the recipient should wrap up warmly after a reflexology massage, especially if it is cold, since tremendous heat can be lost when so relaxed.

General ailments

There are several general ailments that affect differing body parts and, therefore, do not fall into just one of the previous categories. For greater understanding refer to the foot chart on pages 23–4 and then look up the relevant section.

Babies or children mirror the uneasiness of the parents, particularly the mother, so ideally all family members should receive reflexology. As the adults get better, so too do the offspring.

General ailments relieved through reflexology

Regardless of the dis-order, a complete reflexology massage is always required, with specific attention to the:

- nervous system and solar plexus reflexes to calm the mind and relieve any pain, anxiety and fear
- endocrine gland reflexes to soothe the emotions and create inner harmony
- affected gland or organ reflexes to relax the distressed area and ease the symptoms of distress.

Reflexology assists specific ailments in the following ways:

- abscess: accumulated hurts and inflamed emotions surface for eventual release and relief from past traumas
- accidents: dissipates the reckless need to go headlong into situations
- arthritis: replaces rigidity and uncertainty with security and flexibility
- bites: provides protection against perceived outside attack
- blisters: soothes friction that come to a head
- body odour: boosts confidence in oneself
- boils: brings to a head frustrating aspects that have got under the skin
- bruises: eases the emotional knocks in life, using them instead as knocks of opportunity for self-development
- burns: releases extreme anger and frustration that has surfaced
- calluses: removes the need to cover up, protect or conceal true thoughts and emotions, by boosting belief in personal abilities
- cancer: encourages the open expression of true feeling, so that they no longer cause inner havoc and dis-ease
- candida: centres the individual so that they no longer feel frustrated at being pulled in so many directions to please others, but instead nurtures the self for the benefit of all
- carbuncle: releases repressed anger and frustration of life circumstances that get under the skin by coming to a head for complete elimination
- childhood ailments: dismisses the childlike behaviour of adults within the vicinity

- chills: encourages the individual to come in from the cold and to stop withdrawing into the self
- colds: urges mind, body and soul to exonerate outdated belief systems and sad, irritating thoughts to make way for new exciting concepts
- congestion: relaxes the musculature letting go of congested emotions, so that there is a free flow and distribution of energy and enthusiasm throughout the whole
- corns: removes the perceived need to protect personal concepts from being trampled on
- cramp: eases gripping fear
- cuts: creates inner peace so that there is no longer a feeling of being cut up and torn apart
- cysts: eliminates the need to gain attention and recognition of accumulated hurts and injured feelings
- eczema: calms the emotional turmoil of irritants that erupt under the skin
- fatigue: fills the whole with an enthusiasm for life that defies boredom and tiredness
- fever: encourages heated emotions to surface and dissipate
- fever blisters: increases tolerance to heated emotions that cause friction
- fibroid cysts: relaxes the tight grip on accumulated hurts, allowing them to escape and disappear
- fistula: dissipates the need to form emotional escape routes
- fungi: refuses to allow old emotions to dwell and hurt the body
- gangrene: eliminates morbid thoughts and restores faith in the need to be alive
- glandular disorders: enhances the distribution of lively thoughts and ideas for the well-being of the whole
- gout: dismisses the burning need to dominate, replacing anger and impatience with lenience
- infection/inflammation: soothes inflamed, infuriating emotions
- influenza: disposes of mass negativity and beliefs that cause widespread pain and irritability
- itching: meets the innate desire to move ahead or escape from irritating circumstances
- multiple sclerosis: dissolves the strictness of having to conform to rigid belief systems

- muscular disorders: facilitates moving ahead with ease
- nail biting: removes anxiety of having to put one's own ideas into practice by restoring confidence and faith in oneself
- numbness: fills the whole with renewed sensitivity and unconditional love for the self and others
- oedema: expels old emotions that weigh heavily on the mind, body and soul
- pain: banishes the hurt of inadequacy or criticism
- parasites: sets free those who are perceived to be drawing on personal resources
- plantar wart: dissipates frustration and anger about the direction of life
- rheumatism: dissolves past resentment and bitterness
- sclerosis: liberates the whole from an intense desire to control
- shingles: relinquishes the hurt at the inadequacy of putting personal ideas into action
- skin disorders: pacifies the whole so that life does not get under the skin
- snoring: frees deep-seated emotions that have been kept close to the chest
- spinal curvature: reinforces the support and backing
- swelling: liberates entrapped emotions
- twitching: boosts self-esteem and self-confidence by removing anxiety and fear of the consequences
- ulcers: reinstates belief in the self
- warts: removes the need to project concepts of self-hate and ugliness
- weakness: provides inner strength to enjoy the fullness of life
- wounds: heals emotional hurts.

conclusion

Reflexology today and in the future

Reflexology, once valued as a healing medium, became less popular during the scientific revolution around 250 years ago. Like many other concepts that linked the mind, body and soul, it was dismissed as unscientific. The body then became treated as some kind of sophisticated machine that could only be serviced and maintained by highly trained, specialized personnel and equipment.

With armour-plated defence mechanisms and mass belief conditioning it was inevitable that dis-ease and unrest would become widespread. The resultant panic and hysteria worldwide arises from having lost touch with our true selves, as well as with the abundance of the universe.

Boredom, emptiness and world-weariness are symptoms of materialism that impoverish the mind, body and soul. Masses are starved and deprived of a deeper meaning to life that cannot be discovered through systematic, scientific research.

Increasing desperation, from the realization that complete solutions are not available in the physical world alone, has generated renewed interest in ancient healing practices, such as reflexology. Many turn to these ancient forms of healing when all else have failed and are amazed at their effectiveness.

The trend to look for other points of view is expanding with the discovery that inner peace and harmony are possible, even in these distressing times of violence, confusion and fear. More people are taking responsibility for their health and well-being, and in so doing are healing the world through healing themselves naturally.

Reflexology liberates individuals from self-imposed restrictions and encourages people to step ahead to a more fulfilling and meaningful way of life.

There is inside us, all of the potential that we wish to be,
All the energy to do whatever we would like to do,
If we imagine ourselves as we would like to be,
Doing what we wish to do,
And every day take a step towards our dream,
Although at times it may seem impossible
To hold onto that dream,
One day we shall awake
To find that we are the person that we dreamed of,
Doing what we wish to do,
Simply because we had the courage
To believe in our potential,
And hold onto our dream!

May all your dreams come true!

taking it further

Further research

The author, Chris Stormer, is a world acclaimed authority on reflexology. Her previous books are enjoyed by those with a general interest in this fascinating form of healing and are also used as text and hand books in Reflexology and Healing Establishments and Training Centres throughout the world. To supplement the information in this book obtain a copy of:

Reflexology – The Definitive Guide 0 340 62038 2

This book, published by Hodder & Stoughton, London, is available through most literary outlets. If sold out and therefore not immediately available, ask the bookstore to place an order for you.

Reflexology videos, audio tapes and a comprehensive range of foot charts are also available from the author.

Healing enhanced through the use of aromatherapy oils

The sensuous aspect of aromatherapy oils has a therapeutic effect on mind, body and soul. A mixture of one to three oils with approximately 30 ml of almond oil can be rubbed into the feet during or at the end of the massage to enhance the effect of reflexology.

uplifting oils To boost confidence, ease depression and eliminate moodiness. Examples are clary sage, jasmine and grapefruit.

regulating oils To relieve anxiety and re-establish equilibrium. Examples are bergamot, frankincense, geranium and rose-wood.

stimulating oils To strengthen concentration, clear the mind and improve memory. Examples are lemon, peppermint, rosemary and black pepper.

invigorationg oils To fill the whole with enthusiasm and interest and strengthen the immune system. Examples are cardamom, juniper, rosemary and lemongrass.

soothing oils To increase levels of tolerance, improve sleep patterns and calm the mind. Examples are camomile, lavender, marjoram and orange blossom.

aphrodisiac oils To strengthen relationships and boost self-esteem. Examples are jasmine, clary sage, patchouli and ylang ylang.

There are many other valuable aromatherapy oils that can be used to accelerate healing. Specialized books are filled with a wealth of information on the subject.

The vibration of colours for inner harmony

Visualization of colours during reflexology massage alters the vibrational tone of healing energies absorbed by the body. The resultant fine tuning reconnects mind, body and soul for overall harmony and peace.

The following guide recommends colours that can be visualized during reflexology massage of the various areas on the feet. Should another colour come to mind, or if the colour changes, stay with the adjustment since this is the vibration required.

Red on the heels provides security, mobility and enthusiasm for individual growth and development. 'See red' when obstacles are perceived to obstruct personal actualisation.

Orange on the lower insteps communicates the joy at feeling secure within relationships, thereby making life pleasurable.

Yellow on the upper insteps re-establishes control knowing that, with stability and affinity, actions benefit all those concerned.

Green on the balls of the feet harmonizes internal and external relationships with personal achievements, interactions and security, enhancing pure love for oneself and others.

Blue on the toe necks calms and clarifies the mind and body for the open and honest expression of the soul.

Purple on the toes raises the level of consciousness for clarity of thought, peace of mind, emotional harmony and overall body alignment.

Music to relax body, mind and soul

The abundance of beautiful music available today makes it impossible to mention it all, especially when taking into consideration, personal preferences. Here are a few suggestions:

- Dolphin and whale music, especially beneficial for pregnancy and childbirth and for restless or disturbed souls.
- Natural sounds such as the wind, sea, waterfalls, birdsong and so on. Examples:
  - *Wilderness* by Tony O'Connor
  - *Wetland Symphony* by Ducks Unlimited Canada.
- Ethnic music using traditional instruments. Examples:
  - *Cusco, Apurimac II. Return to ancient America*
  - *Eagle* by Medwyn Goodall
  - *Uluru* by Tony O'Connor.
- Pan flutes. Example:
  - *In Touch* by Tony O'Connor.
- Electrical harp. Examples:
  - *Dream Spiral* by Hilary Stagg.
- Other suggestions:
  - *Gifts of the Angels* by Steven Halpern
  - *Bushland Dreaming* by Tony O'Connor
  - *Rhythmist; Inner Tides; Lunar Reflections* by Ian Cameron Smith.

Contacts, reflexology centres and training organizers

Author

Chris Stormer
Tel/fax: +27 (0) 11 803 9052
Email:
inspired@worldonline.co.za
Website: www.alwaysb.com

Reflexology book list

(Larkin's Reflexology Booklist – most comprehensive reflexology booklist)
Website: http://homepage.
eircom.net/~footman

International Holistic Therapists Directory

Geoffrey Keyte
Tel: +353 (0) 51 422209
Email: info@astraldelta.com
Website:
www.internationalholistictherapies.
com

International Reflexology Magazine

Russell McAllister
Reflexology World Magazine
Tel: +61 (0) 2 9300-9391
Fax: +61 (0) 2 9300-9216
Email: reflexworld@pobox.com
Website:
www.reflexologyworld.com

America

Denver
Adrianne L. Fahey
Associated Reflexologists
Colorado
P.O. Box 697
Englewood, CO 80151

Massachusetts
Margo Dussault
Tel: +1 (0) 401 423 1575
Email:
mdu7058u@postoffice.un.edu

Washington State
Shellie Earley
Tel: +1 (360) 833 9899
Fax: +1 (360) 335 1044
Email: feet2reflex@aol.com
Washington Reflexology
Association
Website:
www.washingtonreflexology.org

Australia

Adelaide
Sue Ramsey
Tel/fax: +61 (0) 8 8664 1819
Email: sjramsey@tell.net.au

Brisbane
Catherine Pretorius
Tel/fax: +61 (0) 73 201 0680
Email: cdpre@hotmail.com

Melbourne
Dee Leamon
Tel/Fax: +61 (0) 3 9882 6275
Email: asm@alphalink.com.au

Perth
Joan Cass
Tel/fax: +61 (0) 89 457 3117

Sydney
Sue Ehinger
Tel: +61 (0) 2 4976-3881
Fax: +61 (0) 2 4976-3880
Email: arstraining@aol.com

Canada

Vancouver
Joy Burrows
Salt Spring Island
Tel: +1 (0) 250 537 8411
Email: stmarylake@telus.net
Website: www.innerjoy.ca

Egypt
Rawya El Gammal
Tel: +20 (0) 2 340 3223
Fax: +20 (0) 2 341 1018
Email: sacha@mist-net.com

England

Kent
Salvina Macari
Tel: + 44 (0) 184 3 29 5910
Email: ben.macari@virgin.net

Norfolk
Angela Sellens Drake M.A.R.
Tel: + 44 (0)1603 503794
Email: angelasd@beeb.net

Greece
Rena Stravelaki
Tel: +30 (0) 1 984 1030
Fax: +30 (0) 1 988 0310
Email: lambross@usa.net

Holland
Wilma Meijer
Tel/fax: +31 (0) 72 532 1615
Email: w-meijer@hetnet.nl

Hong Kong
Jean Hudson
Tel: +852 (0) 2358 8295
Fax: +852 (0)2719 9621
Email: gujean@ust.hk

Ireland

Kerry
Angelika Scheibein
Email: gscheibein@hotmail.com

Galway
Marguerite Brady
Tel: +353 (0) 91 634 591
Email: yourmystar@eircom.net

Japan

Miki Tanaka
Email:
myousokusin@hotmail.com

New Zealand

Hamilton
Jeanne van Kuyk
Tel: +64 (0) 7 884 8555
Fax: +64 (0) 884 9494
Email: jjvankuyk@xtra.co.nz

Wellington
Emma Frommings
Tel: +64 (0) 4 239 9421
Fax: +64 (0) 4 239 9433.
Email:
emmafrommings@paradise.net.nz

Scotland

Aberdeen
Helen Young
Tel: +44 (0) 1224 704887

Edinburgh
Di Scott
Tel: +44 (0) 131 661 4150
Email: Diinfeet@aol.com

Glasgow
Sarah-Fiona Helme
Tel: +44 (0) 1698 792551
Email: sarahfionah@yahoo.com

South Africa

Cape Town
Andrea Meyer
Tel: +27 (0) 21 674 0267
Email: madfoam@intekom.co.za

Durban
Yavanee Singh
Tel/fax: +27 (0) 31 312 0881
Email:
yaraka@freemail.absa.co.za

Johannesburg
Keith McFarlane
Tel: +27 (0) 11 682 3584
Email: THC@global.co.za

United Kingdom

General Organiser
Di Scott
Tel: +44 (0) 131 661 4150
Email: Diinfeet@aol.com

Wales

Carmarthenshire
Stephanie Jones
Tel: +44 (0) 1559 371 511
Email:
malindi_centre@v21mail.co.uk
Website: www.malindi.co.uk

Pembrokeshire
Liz Evans
Tel: + 44 (0) 1834 871 402.
Fax: + 44 (0) 1646 690 262
Email: dream90900@aol.com

index